MW01599113

first edition

Published in 2011 by Cat Smiley Books. This book may be purchased for sales and educational use. For information, please write to Suite 618, 106-4368 Main St, Whistler, B.C., V0N 1B4, Canada.

This book is the official workout of *The Original Boot Camp*, used for participants within the healthy weight range. This workout is also used at *Cat Smiley Fat Camp* when participant ability permits. To join, visit www.originalbootcamp.tv or www. fatcamp.tv. To book Cat Smiley for a speaking engagement,

email cat@originalbootcamp.tv

Author: Cat Smiley

Designer: Emma Moldrich

Photographers: Jenna-Mae Togado (cover and back profile), Bonny Makarewicz (boot camp action images, success stories and exercise demonstrations), Darby Magill pages 54, 65, Thomas Smiley 56, 63

Editor: Stefanie Hostetter

ISBN-13: 978-1466274334

ISBN-10: 1466274336

© Cat Smiley 2011. All rights reserved. All content including but not limited to texts, images, concept, and creative arrangement is protected by copyright. No part of this publication may be reproduced, stored in a retrieval system or transmitted in any form or by any means; electric, mechanical, photocopying or otherwise without the written permission of the publisher.

how to
exercise

8 week boot camp modelled by real life beginner client, Erica Cuthbert

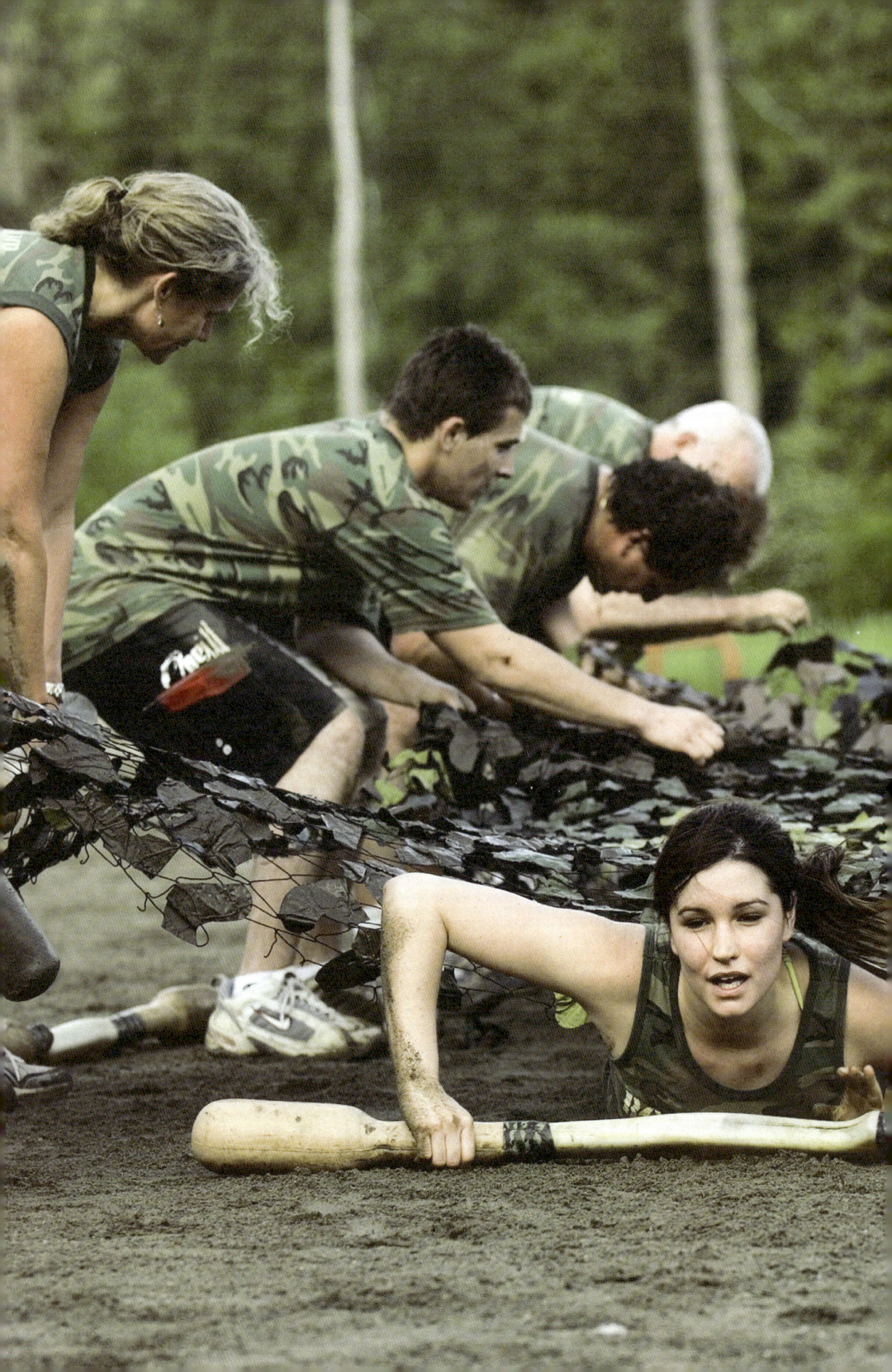

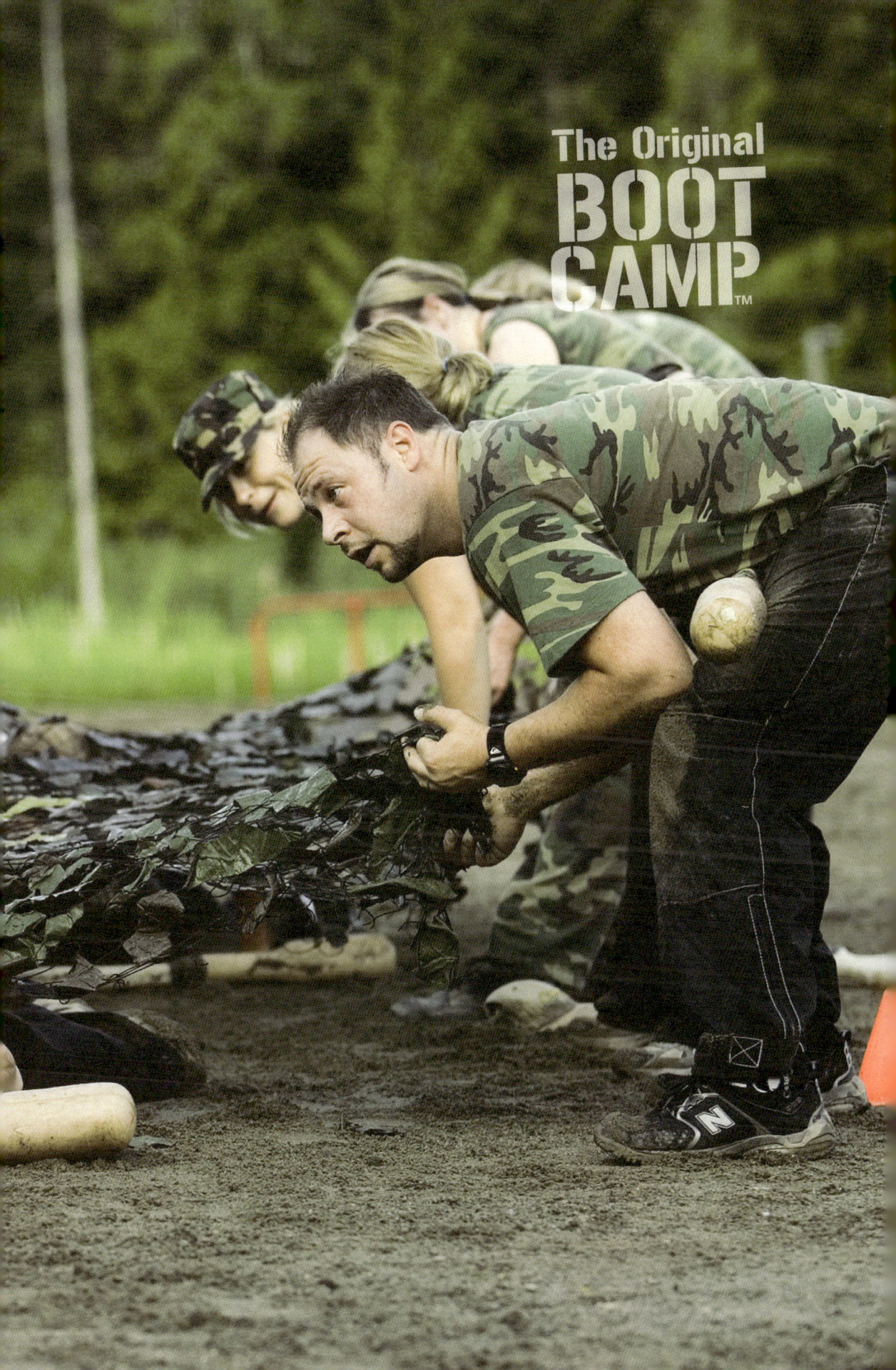

The Original
BOOT
CAMP™

contents

part 1

how to play boot camp

part 2

24 kick ass workouts

part 3

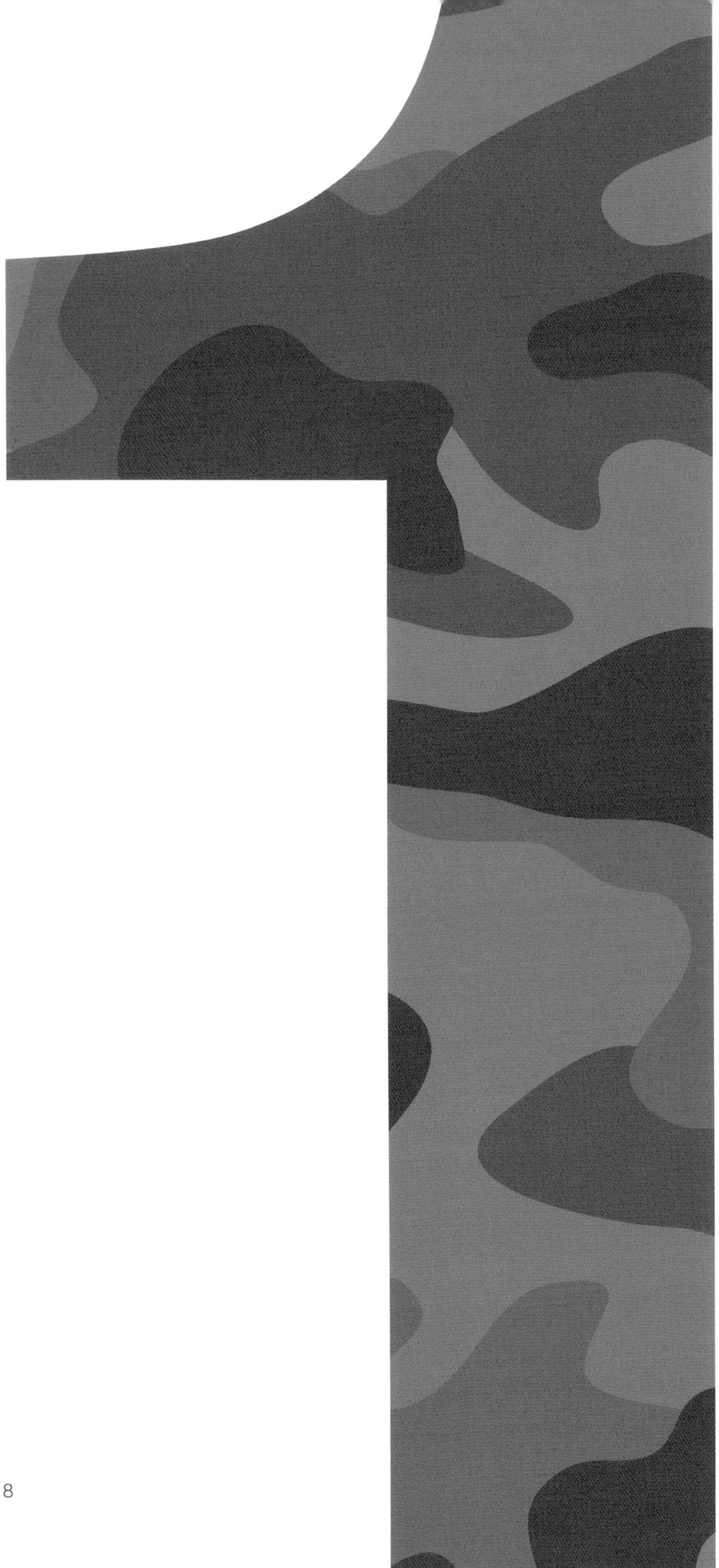

how to play boot camp

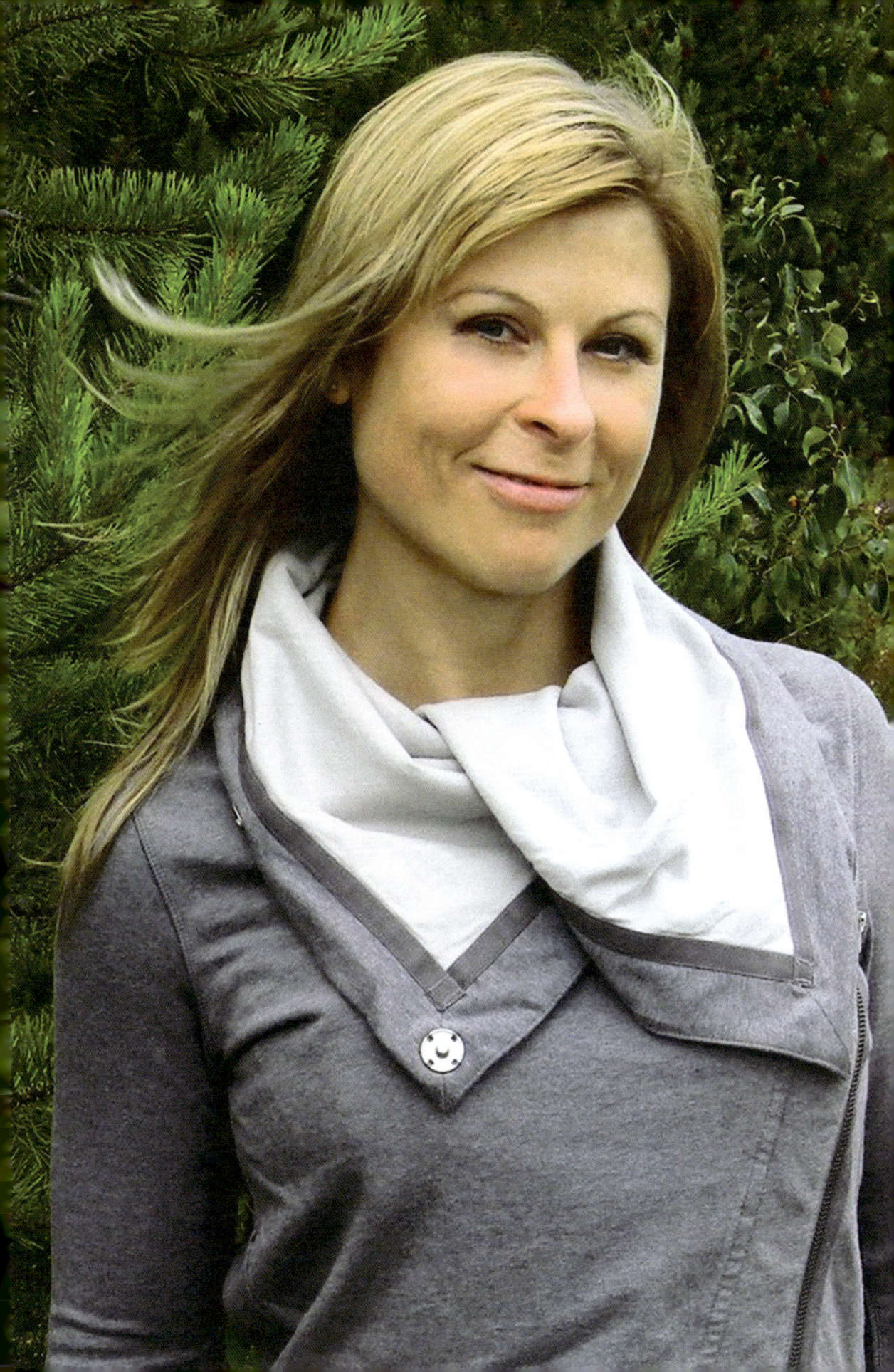

hey team!

I'm so excited to have you here with me, training in the same system that has pioneered the nations hottest fitness trend! *The Original Boot Camp* has a proud history of changing lives and elevating people's perception of what they can achieve.

Although there are a few different levels of ability demonstrated in these workouts, I highly recommend slimming down to within 30lbs of your healthy weight range first, and having a base level of base fitness. Save this workout for when you can run one mile on the treadmill in 12 minutes or less, and do one pushup without going onto your knees. Get your head in the right place to really commit to the program and sticking with it. Find the courage to push your personal limits and believe in something beyond what you previously thought possible. Stay true to yourself and what you know is right - it takes integrity to get real with the fact that there really are no excuses. If a sporty girl like me can sit down and write 3 big books, you can do anything! See it, believe it... do it!

The next 8 weeks of **kick ass workouts** will give you total body transformation and push your personal limits. It's going to be awesome. Go at your own pace and choose the most convenient location - this workout can be done anywhere.

Our training program will include cycles with blocks of endurance and moderate resistance, tapping into your white muscle fibers to increase tone without adding bulk. This combination of fast and slow gives you rapid results and dramatic body composition changes, as you reach the highest athletic training threshold, with minimal risk of injury. It's not going to be easy, your muscles will scream at you, but you know it's time to do this!

The Original Boot Camp is held at the crack of dawn, 5 days a week in all weather conditions....sounds hardcore, but beginners are usually the first ones to sign up. Recruits sprint up hills, do push-ups in the snow, jump logs, chin-ups, pump weights and perform rigorous abdominal training. I take on a tough-as-nails drill sergeant persona, empowering ordinary people to reach extraordinary heights. It's such a buzz - so incredibly exciting and rewarding to see how proud my clients are to be able to do this. It just feels good to kick ass, and be all you can be. Thats why I'm so excited to share my system with you - I just know you're going to love it. Well, it's a love-hate relationship, but in an hour it's all over....before most people are even getting out of bed.

Okay! Let's do this!

Ready?

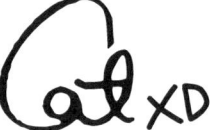

"Cat Smiley is the owner of Canada's first and longest running fitness boot camp, with her innovative system paving the way for others to follow. She is without a doubt the nations pioneer of fitness boot camp trends."~*CBC Radio*

"Declare victory on the battle of the bulge with this boot camp workout! Cat Smiley's charges know her rules: no yelling and no crybabies. It sounds like an episode of *Nanny 911*, but Smiley isn't some militant Mary Poppins"~*Chatelaine Magazine*

"Cat unapologetically pushes clients to the edge of their limits. As Canadian Trainer of the Year for the past 3 years, she brings training back to basics. Her Drill Sergeant style of training has sent Smiley soaring to the top, and people are more than willing come along for the ride."~*Fitness Business Canada*

"The goal isn't to ship out for military service. With the body confidence, functional fitness and renewed motivation that comes from this workout, recruits can focus instead on kicking butt in their outdoor endeavors."~*Explore Magazine*

fitness preparation

Having a base fitness level before doing this workout program is essential, as is being within the healthy weight range.

If you are 30lbs or more overweight, before doing anything you must book your medical evaluation to obtain clearance to begin an exercise program. They will check both your heart rate and blood pressure to determine what state your cardiovascular system is in, and if exercise will place you at risk, plus family history. These are key indicators as to your ability to start exercise and your initial intensity.

For those just starting, water exercise is the best option to get your heart rate up without producing impact on your joints. If you feel insecure in a bathing suit, call the local pool facility to find out the quietest time. You will love the freedom of movement in water that allows the joints to move naturally - the weightlessness makes water non-injurious and therapeutic to the joints. Range of motion and flexibility will also benefit. Combining cardiovascular endurance and strength training using body resistance with a low fat diet, will make you reach your happy size in no time... burning extra calories both during the workout and after.

Knowing the shape of your feet is important and the gait of your running style. Speak with a specialist who can analyze both your feet and gait. They will recommend a brand of shoe, or foot beds to ensure no damage is done. During running the pressure on your joints is 3-4 times your bodyweight compared to if you were walking, so proper support is crucial. Strengthening your connective tissues will decrease the risk of injury and prepare you for unrestricted training and maximum results.

Beginner Cardio Options

(stay in your target zone for about 50min).

- Get good running shoes
- Spend at least two days before you start exercising drinking two litres of water/day.
- Training Heart Rate should stay between 93 – 120 beats per minute.
- Never work harder than 130 beats per minute.
- Record every session in a note book.

Walking

Intervals (pace should be based on Heart Rate).

- 1 mile warm-up at a slow pace then stretch the lower body for 5 minutes.
- ¼ mile at slow pace.
- ¼ mile at medium pace.
- ¼ mile at slow pace.
- 1 mile at fast pace.

Step ups

Use a step (bench or box) that is approximately mid shin height. From here stand with both feet together and step up onto the box finishing with both feet on-top of the box, ensure the whole foot is on the box. Step back off of the box, and repeat using the other leg as the lead leg and alternate legs.

Elliptical

Mix up fat burning and x-training mode to a maximum of 60 minutes, slow pace. Keep your heart rate monitor at all times and stay below 120bpm.

Treadmill

Incline Intervals – warm-up slow pace 2mph for 10 minutes then take 5 minutes to stretch. Use a comfortable speed, adjusting incline every few minutes. As you progress, start at a higher incline and go faster. Just be sure to keep your heart rate below 130 beats per minute, which is at a level that is still comfortable to talk.

Recumbent Stationary Bike

- Mix up random and hill mode to a maximum of 60 minutes, slow pace.
- Keep your heart rate monitor at all times and stay below 120 beats per minute.
- Progression: Start at comfortable RPM, aim to keep the same pace for the entire session. Every 4 weeks aim to increase your RPM.

X-Training Cardio

- 5 minutes warm-up on the treadmill, followed by 5 minutes lower body stretching
- 10 minutes Elliptical
- 10 minutes Rower
- 10 minutes Stationary Bike
- 10 minutes Treadmill cool-down (no incline)

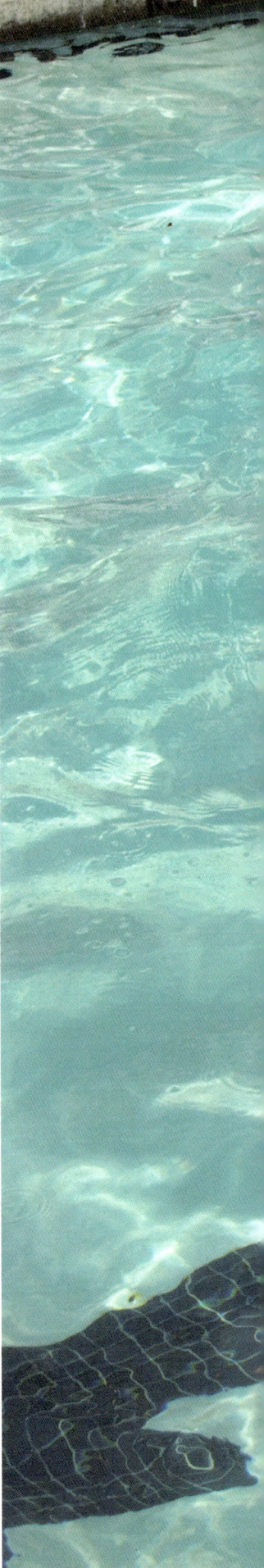

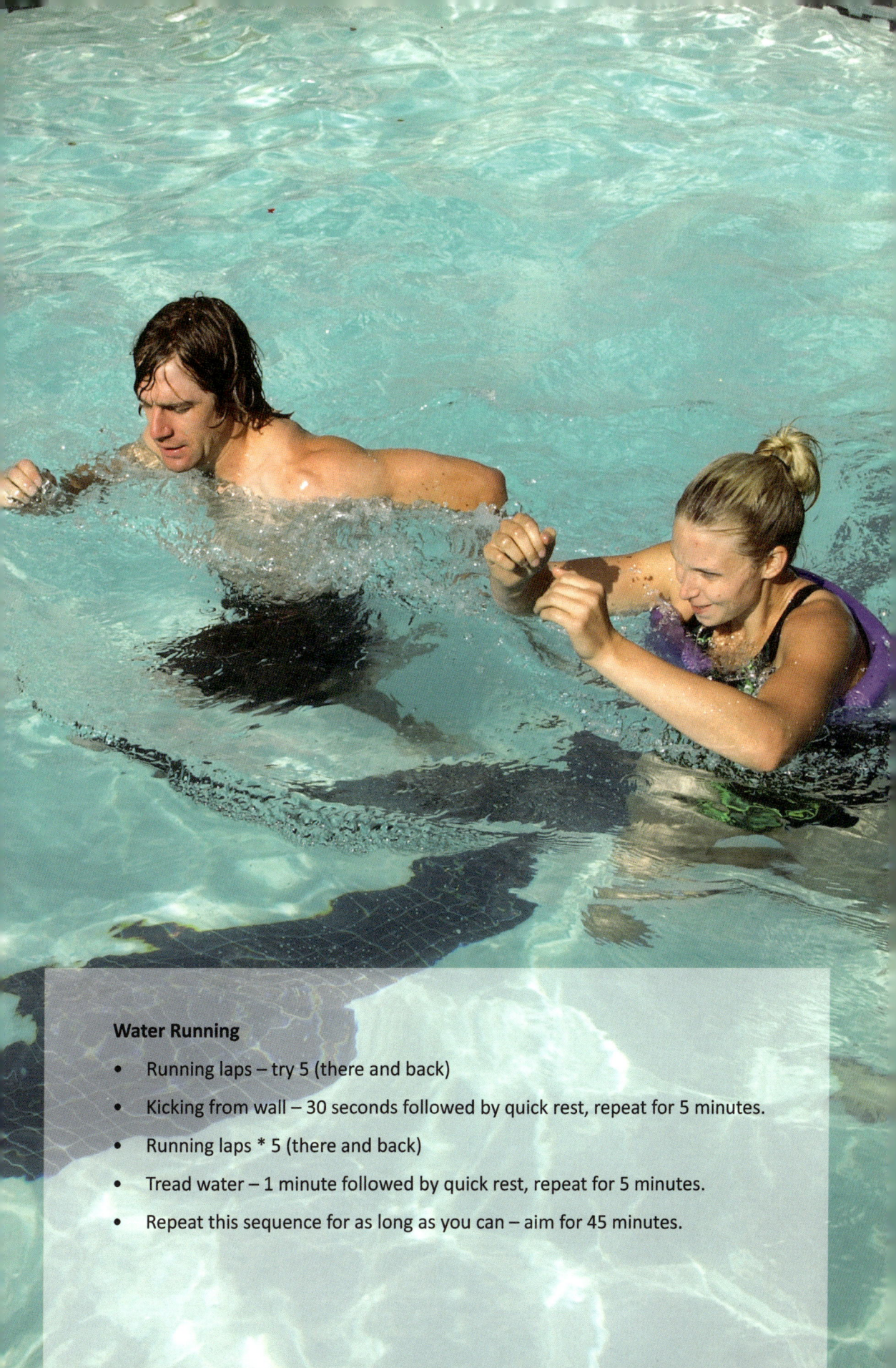

Water Running

- Running laps – try 5 (there and back)

- Kicking from wall – 30 seconds followed by quick rest, repeat for 5 minutes.

- Running laps * 5 (there and back)

- Tread water – 1 minute followed by quick rest, repeat for 5 minutes.

- Repeat this sequence for as long as you can – aim for 45 minutes.

gear list

1 stop watch

2 dumb bells - most recruits buy a set of 5, 7 or 10lbs, and a single 12lb.

3 yoga mat

4 good outdoor running shoes

Check out **www.originalbootcamp.tv** and get into the boot camp mood!

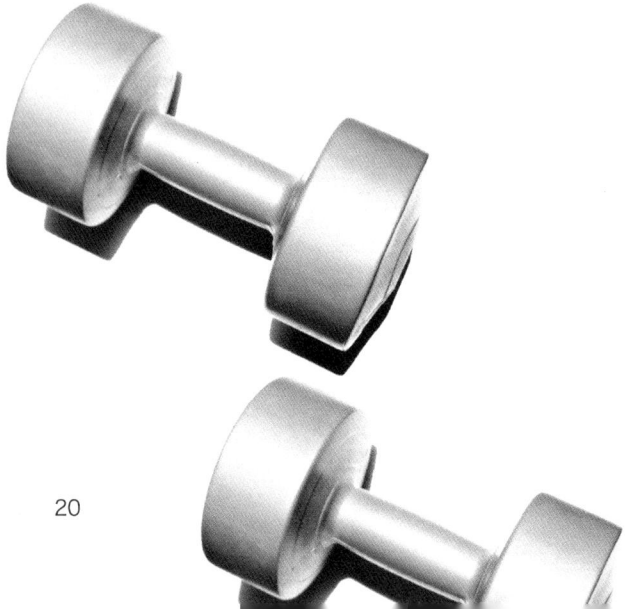

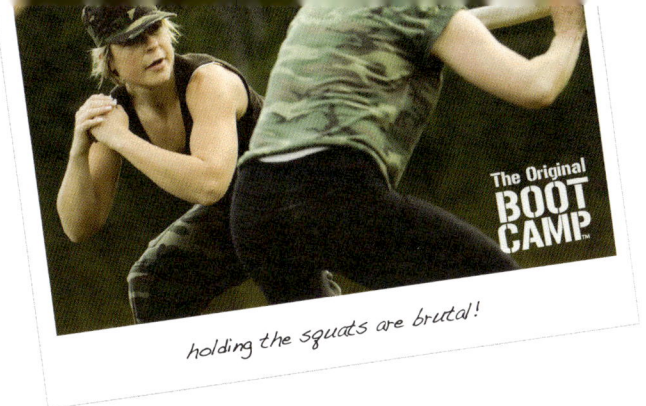

holding the squats are brutal!

survival tactics

1. How should I prepare for our sessions?

The first thing you need to do is get your nutrition sorted. Don't start training until you're properly hydrated - if you've come from not drinking much water at all, it will take about a week of drinking 2 liters a day to get your hydration level back to the safety zone.

Start slow and build up gradually. The body needs time to adapt to increased stresses – overdoing it will increase chance of injury and hinder the process with us. Walking, jogging, hiking and generally staying active will give you a good base to prepare ligaments and tendons for the increased tension that weight training will place on them. Work up to being able to run a mile in 12 minutes or less on the treadmill - that's when you know that you're ready for this workout.

2. What shoes should I get?

It's important to wear shoes that fit the shape of your feet and the gait of your running style. Go to a running store and get set up by a professional to make sure you get the right brand for your needs. Foot beds can help - running puts 3 to 4 times more pressure on your joints than walking. Good shoes are essential!

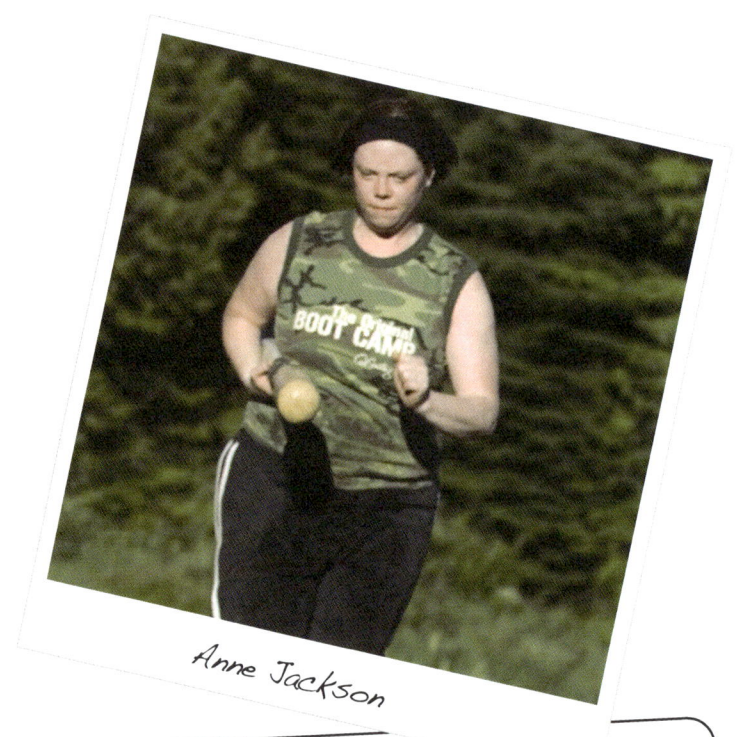

Anne Jackson

anne jackson

At 5'7, 200lbs I was proud to be 'voluptuous, curvy'. I didn't have the desire to change my eating or exercise habits (nor did I think I had to). Then I started exercising consistently with The Original Boot Camp™, and can honestly say it improved my life. I am happier, less stressed and have more energy. I eat because I am hungry, not bored. I am confident and safe in my ability to do activities, riding a bike again and playing soccer for the first time. I am excited to exercise and find I am less likely to stay late at work as I want to go for hike, run or bike ride. I have more patience in stressful situations.

I stuck with The Original Boot Camp™ for over a year, and lost 40lbs. My attitude about life has changed. Exercise has helped me maintain personal balance between work and everything else. I am proud of myself that I am able to exercise regularly. I will always be a regular exerciser now....it makes me feel great!!!

There are lots of people out there who think that they are too out of shape to start a group fitness program, and the only thing I can say is that being out of shape is a temporary state - we have to start somewhere. Starting boot camp made me realize how unfair I was being to my body- each day I have a choice; I could either be embarrassed for being out of shape or proud to have the ability and drive to do something about it.

3. *This is hard! How do people get through this?*

Finding the athlete mindset is a key element of starting this training program. You need to want to be the best, and to create an environment that gives you the drive to want to reach these summits. Change your mental approach to exercise and success will follow. Visualization is a common mental technique that athletes use to feel a movement or trigger the beginning of a specific routine. For example, creating (and storing) the mental image of you sprinting up a hill - or wearing a bikini with confidence, can trigger positive emotions that will help you find drive and motivation.

Raise your expectations of what you can achieve - destroy barriers or limitations you had in the past. Don't let anyone, or anything hold you back!

4. *Do girls train differently?*

We aren't born with the athlete traits of strength, power, drive, and aggression, it is something that is cultivated. It usually comes easier for boys to develop these traits, as ambition, confidence, and standing up for yourself are largely considered masculine qualities (*Bem Sex Role Inventory*).

Some girls are raised to be divas while others get down and dirty. Some climb trees, others are afraid of puddles. The bottom line is that we are all different, but kicking ass is something that is defined differently for all of us. For example, if I get up at 5am and go running, it really doesn't matter to me how far or how fast I go. All that matters is that I hauled myself out of bed at 4.30am and actually went.

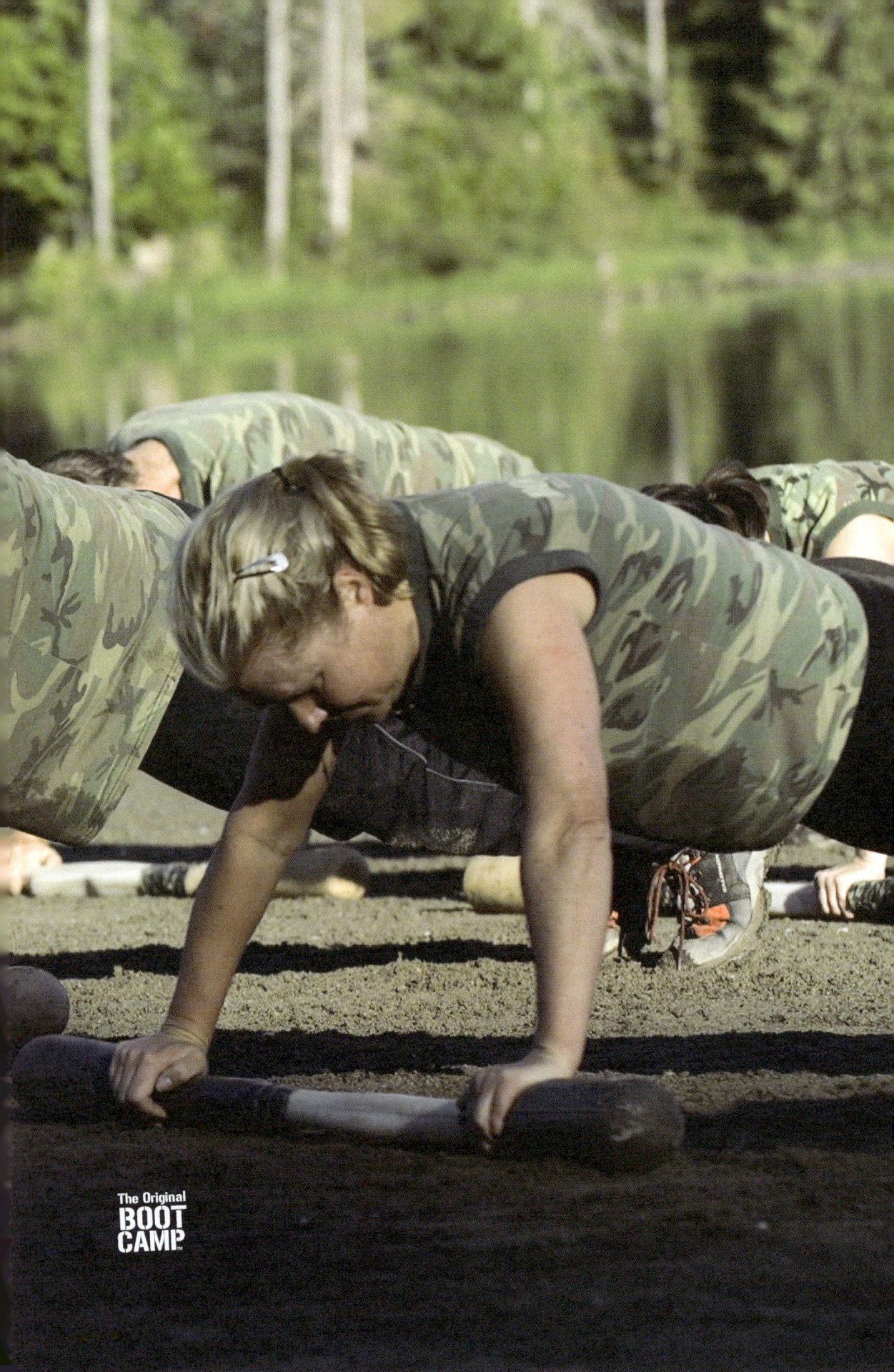

The Original
BOOT
CAMP

Girls don't need to train differently to guys, but sometimes girls need to watch a few re-runs of *Tomb Raider* to be reminded of how kick ass we can be if we are in put in the social environment to do so.

5. What do you consider cardio?

Cardiovascular training refers to the system (heart and lungs) responsible for the uptake and delivery oxygen around the body. In fitness we use this term to describe working our bodies at a level that makes us breathe at a level that is uncomfortable to talk, for about 20 minutes or more. Your heart and breathing rate increase as the demand for oxygen has increased.

6. What should my heart rate be at?

Your heart rate should be around 65-85% percent of your maximum - buy a heart rate monitor to ensure you're training in the right zone. Subtract your age from 220 and multiply it by this percentage to find your zone and stay there for 30 to 90 minutes, at least 3 days a week.

7. Why do we do 25 repetitions?

This is the best way to boost muscle tone while keeping you slim and strong. You can mix up the repetition counts to suit your needs - if you're trying to build bulkier muscle, for example, try working with 5 sets of 12 repetitions.

You should be reaching fatigue for the last few repetitions in the set - this will elicit the targeted muscular adaptation.

8. Will I have sore muscles?

Yes. When you don't exercise for a while, your body will return to a state where being sedentary feels natural. So a sudden return to exercise will cause a shock to the system as you are breaking this balance and stressing the body over and above what it has become used to. The body responds by sending signals of soreness to alert you that it is uncomfortable. Your job is to convince your body that exercising is natural again!

Soreness usually happens due to lactic acid build up. Lactic acid is a by-product of anaerobic glycolysis which happens when you get out of breath as your body can't use oxygen as a fuel to keep it going. It then breaks down glycogen (stored form of glucose) to find energy and keep you going.

Lactic acid is an acid that cripples your muscles ability to maintain training at a high intensity - stopping you from sprinting faster or jumping higher.

Soreness can kick in several days after your workout due to what is known as 'delayed onset of muscle soreness'. This is when you create microscopic tears within the muscle fibers which cause inflammation, forming scar tissue to repair these tears. This is the beginning of the repair phase, and the soreness is often controlled by how much you stretch and walk out this scar tissue.

This microscopic tearing is related to a certain type of muscle contraction which stresses the muscle fibers, called an eccentric contraction. This means that when the muscle is being contracted, it is also being lengthened. This type of contraction is a great way to train due to the stress it places on the muscles and the fast strength gain it results in due to the body being forced to adapt. This soreness is a sign that our training is really working.

jim douglas

Pushing my physical limits at The Original Boot Camp™ helped me be a better father and husband. Stress from everyday life, parenting, work, family, all can contribute becoming lean, but that doesn't mean you're healthy! Since training with Cat, my focus and concentration all have improved. I am also more diligent and determined.

During my time at The Original Boot Camp™ I achieved many personal gains, but most of all, respect. You need confidence to present yourself and gain the respect of others. Finding your limits of physical exercise is one of the most basic traits of human nature.

I have since crossed that boundary of what I thought personally not physically possible, which has been one of the most satisfying moments, and wow, so much changes. Confidence is an amazing word, arguably the most used, yet misunderstood, and underrated cliché in sports. SELF RESPECT is the start of any great personal achievement, and definitely gained at The Original Boot Camp™.

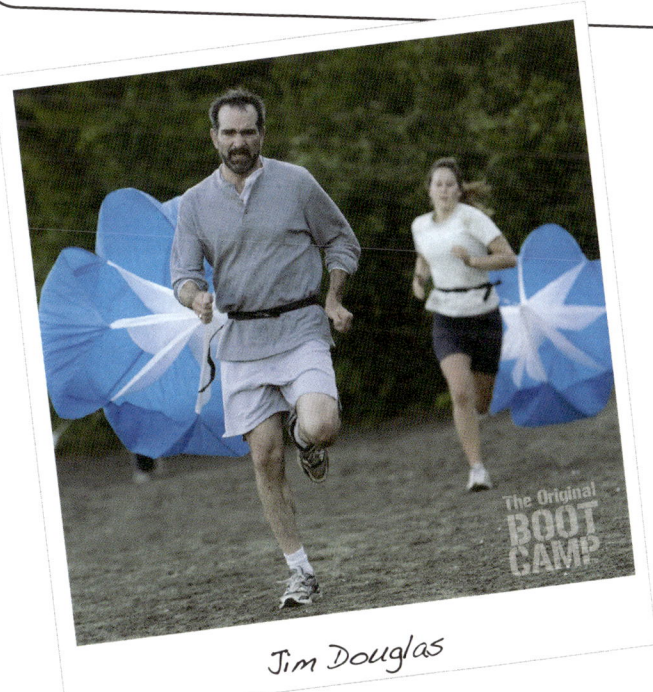

Jim Douglas

9. Why do I feel nauseous?

You may feel dizzy, light-headed and nauseous when you are training hard. Only push to this level if you are an advanced exerciser or you are training with an experienced coach.

What happens to get to this point is that the lactic acid builds in your muscles to a level that brings intense burning pain, being out of breath and elevated heart rate. This is related to the oxygen traveling through your body, and during intense efforts there isn't enough available to continue using the aerobic system to create energy, making you work 'anaerobically'. This is a latin term meaning 'without oxygen'.

When you are working without oxygen your body creates it's energy by switching to glycolysis. This system will work without oxygen supplying energy to the muscles for a few minutes of high intensity effort, depending on your fitness level. The fitter you are, the more you can handle!

Then the burning muscles and 'somebody save me' feelings kick in and you'll have to scale back the intensity back so you can work with oxygen again and breathe easier - for example you may be doing jump squats on a log and you suddenly feel clumsy and dizzy.

All of this is safe, it is simply your body telling you that you've reached a point where it can't keep up with the demands placed on it, so vomiting is a fast way to get rid of the acid build up. Although people usually don't *actually* vomit, some really do feel like they will and what happens at this point depends on your drive, commitment, athleticism and training environment. Make the judgement call when it's time to take a break, and learn your personal limits. Its good to push your comfort zone, but it's important to stay safe.

10. Will weights bulk me up?

No - weight training is about toning, muscle building and strength training. If your goal is to improve your muscular endurance and tone then you will be lifting weights approximately 45-65% of your maximum, between 25-100 repetitions, with several sets (4-5) at a fast tempo, with little rest between exercises. This type of training is often completed as a circuit where exercises are timed and you transition quickly between exercises. This type of training will improve muscle endurance, tone and aid in weight loss.

Building muscle mass is about increasing the size of the muscle fibers. This type of training is intense, requiring weight lifts between 65-85% of your maximum ability, usually doing 3 or 4 sets of 10-12 repetitions at a slow pace (resting a minute between sets).

Strength training again is a further step up. The best way to build strength is to lift between 85-100% of your maximum, 5-6 reps, 1-3 sets with the intent of moving the weight as fast as possible (dependant on goals), with a full recovery between both reps and sets, which is usually around 3-5 minutes.

Women simply don't produce enough testosterone naturally to gain large muscle fiber size unless they follow a very specific type of training.

11. *What is a taper week?*

This is a week when you relax your workouts enough to revamp your enthusiasm for training, and boost results when you come back. The best time to do this is the week before you start your 8 week program, and the week you end it. This will make sure that you're training in the right zone to improve.

When you go back to training, aim to push hard! All your energy stores, muscle fibres, ligaments and tendons will wake up and return to being able to train at an even higher level than before - allowing you to lift more, run faster, or recover quicker than before. This allows you to break through to the next level and kick ass in your workouts...beyond what was possible before.

leanne rodgers

The Original Boot Camp™ feels like an adventure, and starting the day doing something I feel good about makes the rest of my day better. I have become a higher achiever since committing to my training.

The first year I started The Original Boot Camp™, I became the top sales person in my company. I have a greater balance in my life now since my health is not short-changed. I have a greater sense of confidence and can handle the stresses of everyday life better – giving more to my family and work. When it feels hard to get up in the morning I just think get up, go; get it done in an hour! I remind myself that I will have a sense of accomplishment and feel great for the rest of the day.

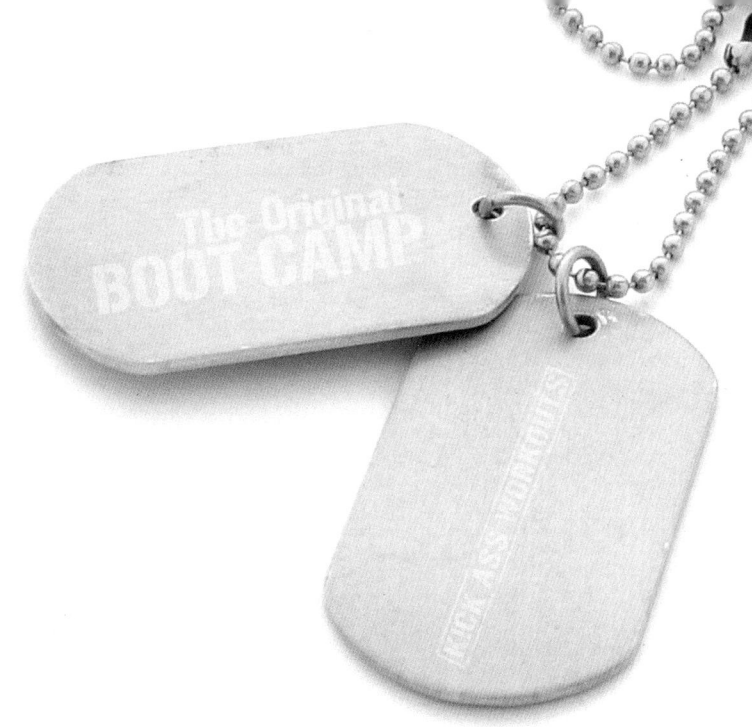

12. When will results kick in?

You'll feel better right away – from the first workout. And after 21 days you'll feel stronger, slimmer and find yourself in the routine of working out.

By the 4 week mark you'll see major changes to the way your body is able to cope with the stresses of working out. Things suddenly seem to get easier around this point, which is when it's a good idea to back off or taper off your cardio a little. During this week, focus on other important elements of your health, such as sleep.

13. Why is rest important?

Muscle tissue repair and growth is very active during rest, recovery and sleep, as is bone re-modeling, reinforcing of ligaments and tendons, the laying down of new cells to replace those that have been damaged through the microscopic tearing that happens when you train hard!

Rest regenerates your energy supplies, leaving you rejuvenated and refreshed. Use your rest time to eat well, explore new recipes and catch up on your social life. Training can wait!

14. How often should we weigh?

Some experts recommend weighing yourself no more than once a week, I recommend every day. This is backed up by research presented at an obesity conference in Vancouver recently that revealed a study showing test groups who weighed daily lost the most weight.

The logic behind this may be that it is easier to catch slight weight gains as they appear, rather than weighing once a month and being face to face with an overwhelming five or ten pound gain. Losing half a pound is a much more attainable goal, and easier to think about making small adjustments to your lifestyle.

Muscle weighs more than fat and everyone's bone density and body is different. Only you know what your best weight is, and when you feel your best. Think of the scale as an incomplete Polaroid of what is really happening with your body as you shape up. The body is up to 75% water, and weight can fluctuate hourly depending on fluid changes, humidity, air pressure, sodium levels, sweating and in response to exercise. It's not uncommon to gain 3lbs from morning to night, and for women, another 5lbs as menstruation approaches. You'll naturally want to eat about 500 calories more before your period, but this will be countered with decreased appetite once it is here. This is why the weight gain is not permanent.

15. Does muscle really weigh more than fat?

A pound of bricks weighs the same as a pound of butter so muscle does not technically weigh more than fat. However muscle is denser than fat and therefore takes up less room in the body, which means that you will weigh more (and likely become a smaller size). Athletic bodies always weigh more than you'd think. The muscular system of the human body consists of about 600 skeletal muscles and account for about 40% of the body's weight. Muscle is 3 times more dense than fat. To lose fat and slim down permanently, you've got to build muscle. The muscle you build will increase your metabolism.

Lean body mass takes more energy to sustain than fat does. Muscle tissue is highly active even when it is resting, whereas fat tissue is comparatively inactive. When you lift weights, you build up lean muscle. Your body will burn 30 to 50 more calories every day for each pound of muscle you put on. As you become more muscular, you become more of a calorie-burning machine. Since weight training is the single most effective manner in which to increase your muscularity, it is a great tool for augmenting the muscle tissue that will automatically burn fat all through the day, even on days you are not working out.

16. Will I gain the weight back?

Carrying extra pounds makes everything that much more difficult, not to mention the extra stress this extra weight is placing on your joints. Keep a strict diet while you're training, to drop excess fat and maximize results.

Exercise boosts many systems operating your body, so if you simply stop, the body will revert back to how it was before. If you stop training: mood and self confidence will drop as exercise releases endorphins which are the 'feel good' chemicals within the brain. Your metabolism won't reach the same peaks as it would if you were exercising. Your cardiovascular system will slowly return to an untrained state, therefore oxygen supply to working muscles will be less efficient.

Exercise also increases HDL (high density lipoprotein) which removes LDL (low density lipoprotein) from artery walls, therefore blood pressure will slowly increase again, which places extra stress on the heart and blood delivery vessels. Reducing your workouts will reduce your immune system efficiency to react and act on any foreign bodies entering the body, making you more vulnerable to getting sick.

17. Why is sleep so important?

Sleep is the time where our bodies gain valuable time to recover, build and adapt to daily stresses placed on it during the day. It is recommended that we get 8 hours sleep a night as this has been researched as the minimum time required for our bodies to recover and adapt in preparation for the next day. However when exercise is in the equation this time often isn't enough as exercise places all systems in an elevated state therefore requiring more energy to run which is very taxing both mentally and physically.

Exercise is known to increase overall energy levels but often makes you sleep more because your body needs more time to recover from the physical stresses put on your body. When you sleep, all your systems return to base level so that is can concentrate on allowing what little energy it is operating on to be used on recovery. Muscle tissue repair and growth is very active during sleep, as is bone remodeling, reinforcing of ligaments and tendons, the laying down of new cells to replace those that have been damaged and discarded, and re-stocking energy stores.

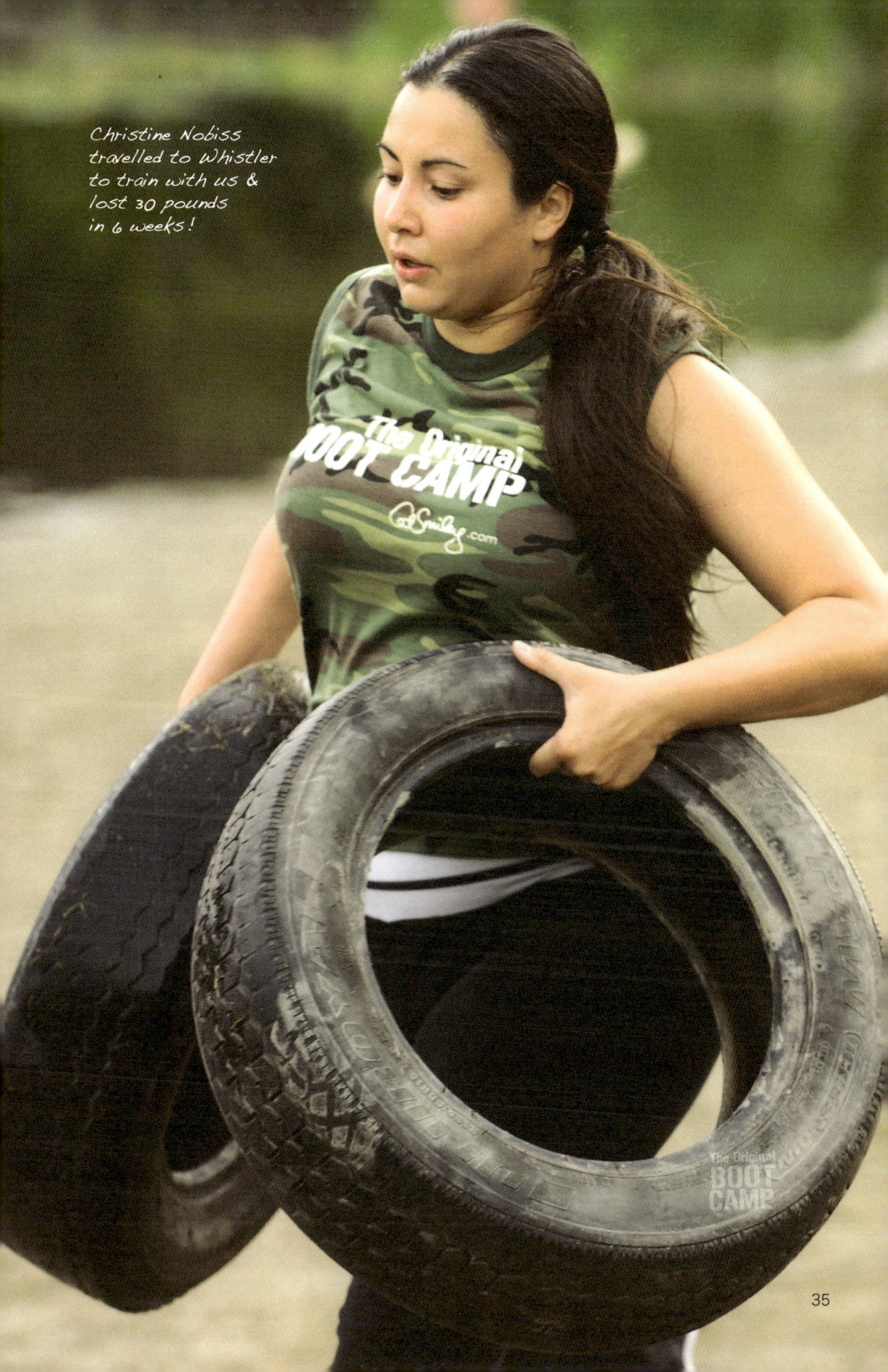

Christine Nobiss travelled to Whistler to train with us & lost 30 pounds in 6 weeks!

18. What should I eat before boot camp?

Trial and error is the best way to figure out what works best for you, but I strongly recommend having at least 150 calories of carbohydrate based fuel before you show up to session. This could be a latte, a piece of toast, or some orange juice....caffeine is a good booster to have before training. When you come back from boot camp, eat within 45 minutes to burn the most calories. I call this the metabolic window, where you should be eating the most balanced meal you possibly can and fueling for the day.

Breakfast needs to be as balanced nutritionally as any other meal. Think quality over quantity, start your day with a good breakfast and mornings will become as high-energy as the rest of the day.

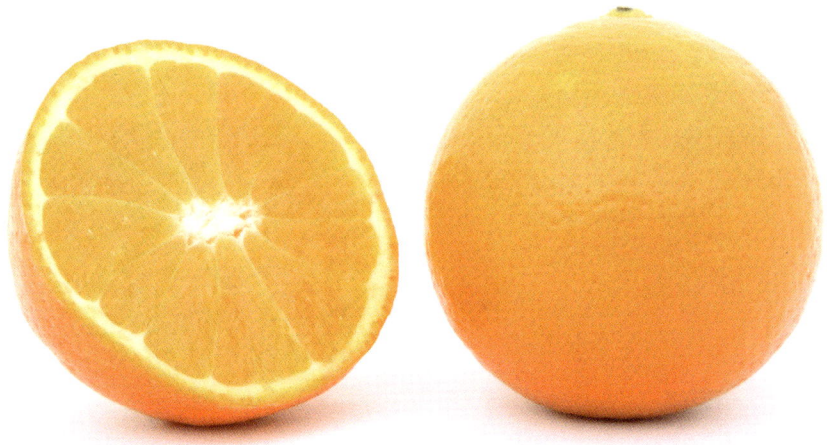

glenn rodgers

If you're going to take time out of your busy schedule to exercise do it like you mean it! The biggest step towards a healthy lifestyle is taking the first one. When I put my fear aside and tried The Original Boot Camp™, I began to feel better physically, which made me stronger mentally as well. I realized that what I did and what I ate really do add up to better health and a better quality life.

I'm motivated by the people I train with at The Original Boot Camp™. I've seen recruits take huge strides in their physical conditioning and appearance, which inspires me to keep pushing and to challenge myself to be better also.
The camaraderie of a group is great because you know that we're all inspired by others accomplishments. When you see someone achieve a standard you thought was impossible you realize that you can get there too with a little more effort.

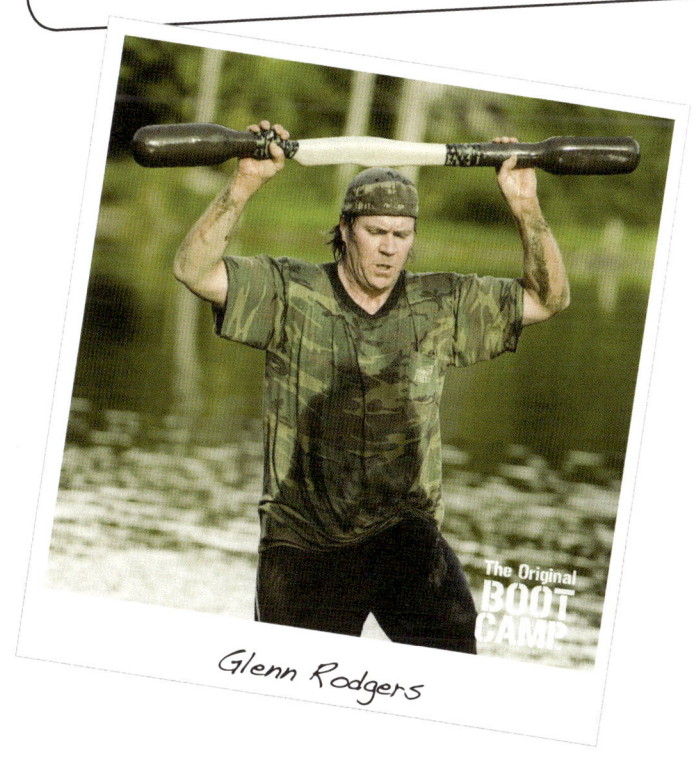

Glenn Rodgers

19. Why is water so important?

Everything in your body needs water to function properly, including breathing, digestion, metabolism, waste removal, and temperature regulation. Water controls many different reactions in your body and is responsible for transportation of nutrients via the blood such as oxygen. And this we can't live without!

People who are overweight, tired or stressed usually have not had enough water. Dehydrated, they can feel tired, sluggish and irritable. Thirsty people often develop extreme cravings for food, misreading the signals their body is sending them to drink water.

Staying hydrated throughout the day is vital for every aspect of your health, from your fat-burning ability to attention span.

clint goyette

Since I joined The Original Boot Camp™ I have found that I have more energy to play with my kids. Kids keep you on the move, but that doesn't build strength or cardio. Even the busiest of kids won't get you up to 80% of your maximum heart rate! That is why a program such as The Original Boot Camp™ is essential for parents who want to increase their fitness and keep up with the kids.

Keeping fit ties into all the other successes of my life. I used to work out all the time - before I had a family, a job and a business. Waking up and seeing a toned body in the mirror acquired from The Original Boot Camp™ makes me feel much better than the out of shape Dad I saw before.

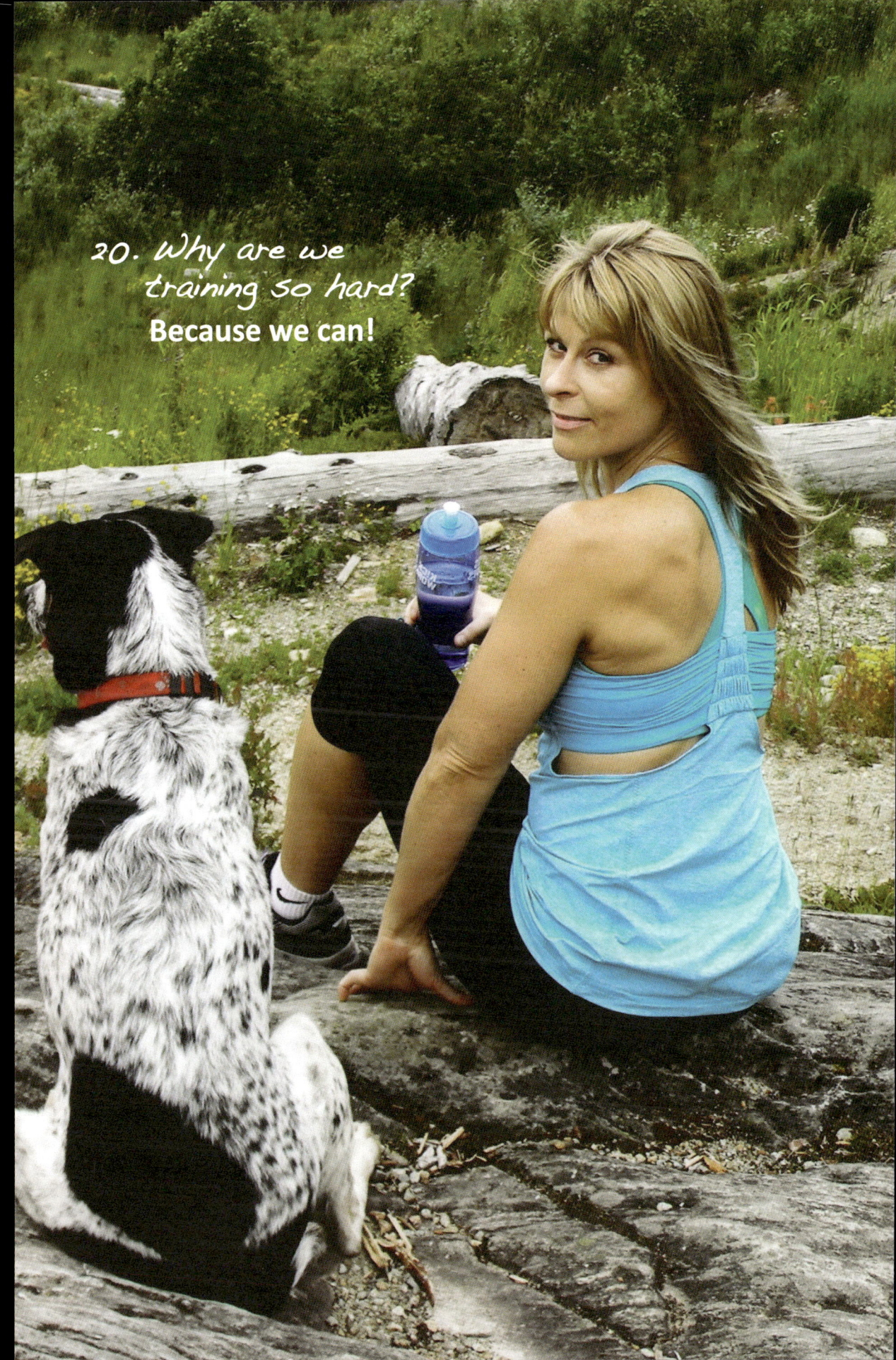

20. Why are we training so hard? Because we can!

erica the boot camp model

This book is all about keeping it real, and what better way than have the exercises modeled by one of my beginner clients?

My goal with Erica was to lose 20lbs in 8 weeks....she lost 35!! We shot the photos for the workout every Monday, and you can see her dramatic transformation week by week.

"I have always struggled with my weight and been extremely self-conscious about it. I never dieted; I would get fit with spurts of fad exercise programs, lose some weight and put it all back on later. When I enlisted in *The Original Boot Camp*, I had just ended a 5 year relationship that kept me unhappy and insecure, with no encouragement to eat well or exercise - it was easier to be overweight. So when we broke up, I knew it was time to finally shape up, but I never thought I would get the results I did!

My only goal on the first day was to get through it. Little did I know that my muscles had completely forgotten how to work that hard. By the next Wednesday I couldn't squat to sit, or go down stairs! I spent a lot of time at night with my legs elevated and wrapped in ice packs. I got up the next morning and the following mornings after that and kept at it, I sweated and huffed and puffed. But I kept telling myself not to quit, even though I thought that lifting a 10lb weight was impossible - and I couldn't run for 3 minutes without stopping.

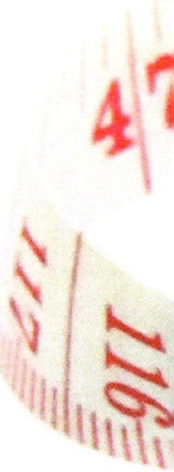

But I stuck with it and went from a size 16 to a size 6, utterly transforming my body and mind. If a 'lifetime chubby girl' like me can do it, so can you! Even if you're an absolute beginner, you can start at any level and move your way up. I recommend it to anyone!!!"

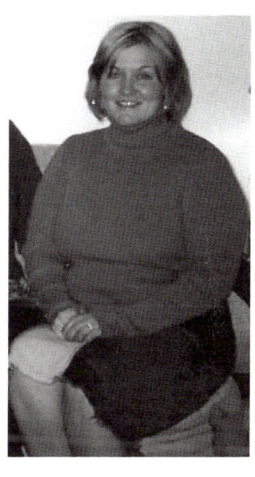

Erica lost **35 lbs** & **29 inches** in 8 weeks!

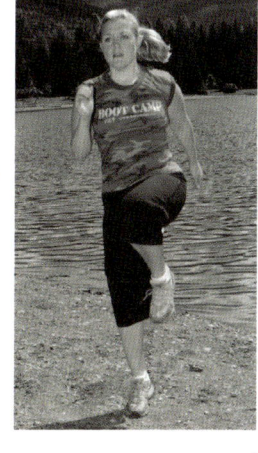

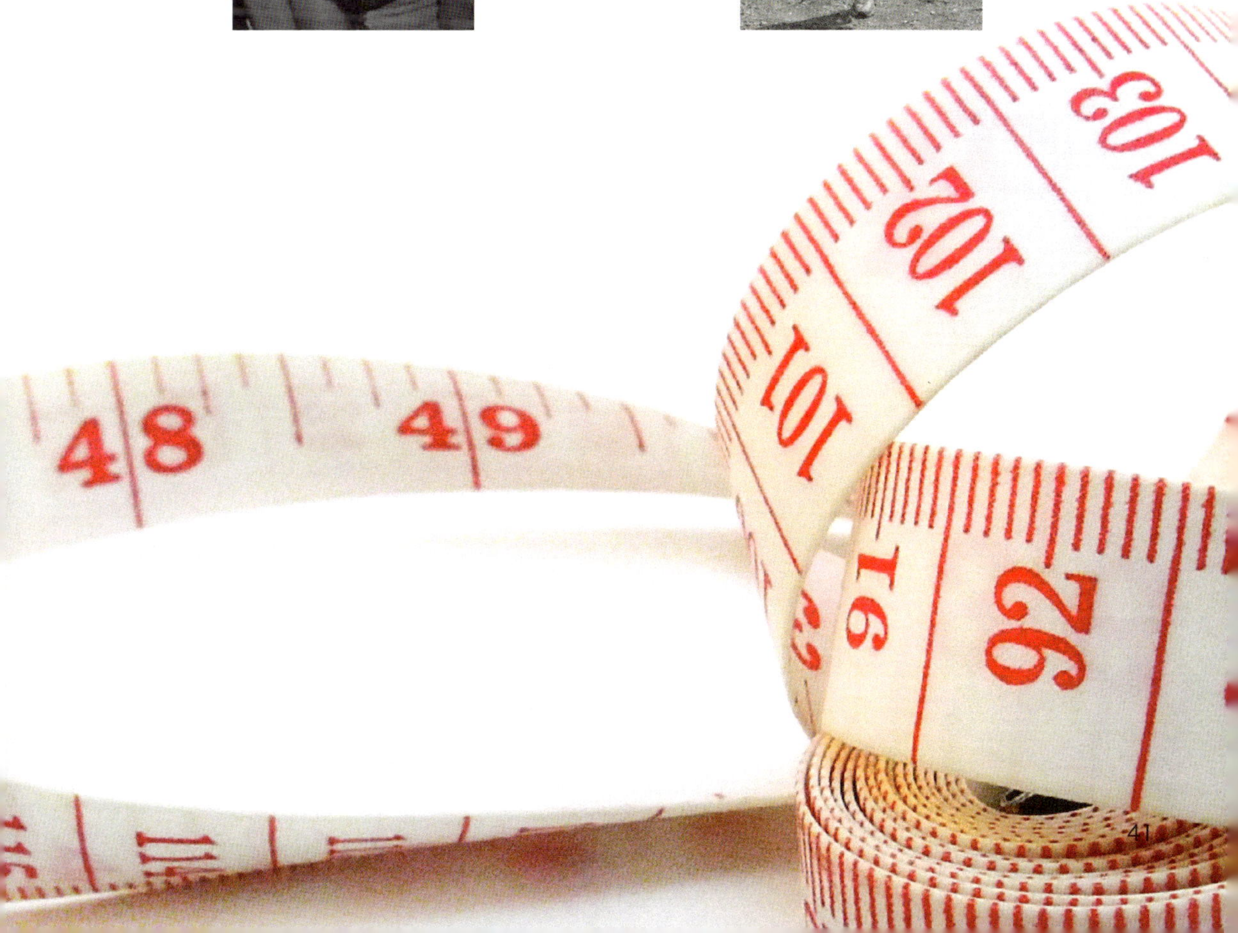

What will your success story be in 8 weeks?

This is your page to write specific, personal goals. Imagine how great you'll feel achieving them! Remember, you are only limited by your patience to stick with it, and dedication to give it your best - all the way to the end.

_____

_____

_____

_____

_____

_____

_____

_____

_____

_____

_____

_____

_____

_____

_____

_____

_____

_____

_____

_____

_____

_____

What will be your biggest challenges?

1. _____

_____

2. _____

_____

3. _____

_____

How will you overcome them?

1. _____

_____

2. _____

_____

3. _____

_____

Ask 3 people to support your boot camp mission, and rat you out should you get back on the pizza-at-midnight wagon.

1. _____

2. _____

3. _____

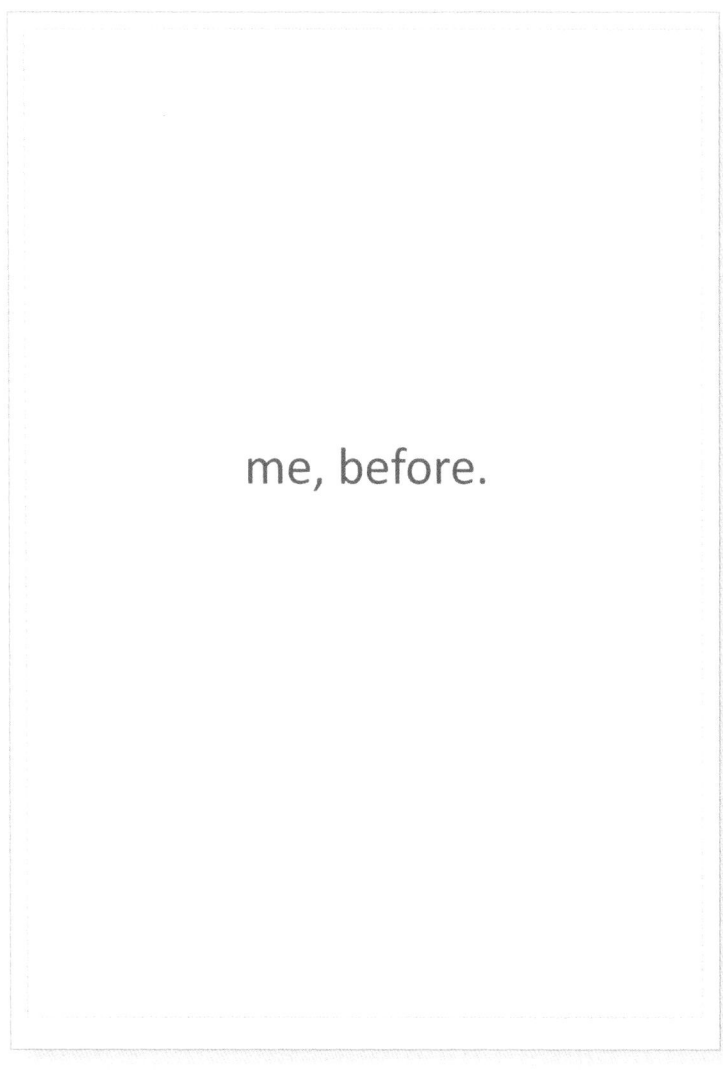

me, before.

weight _____

Face yourself. See the reality of what you look like today and use
this as motivation to transform this image.

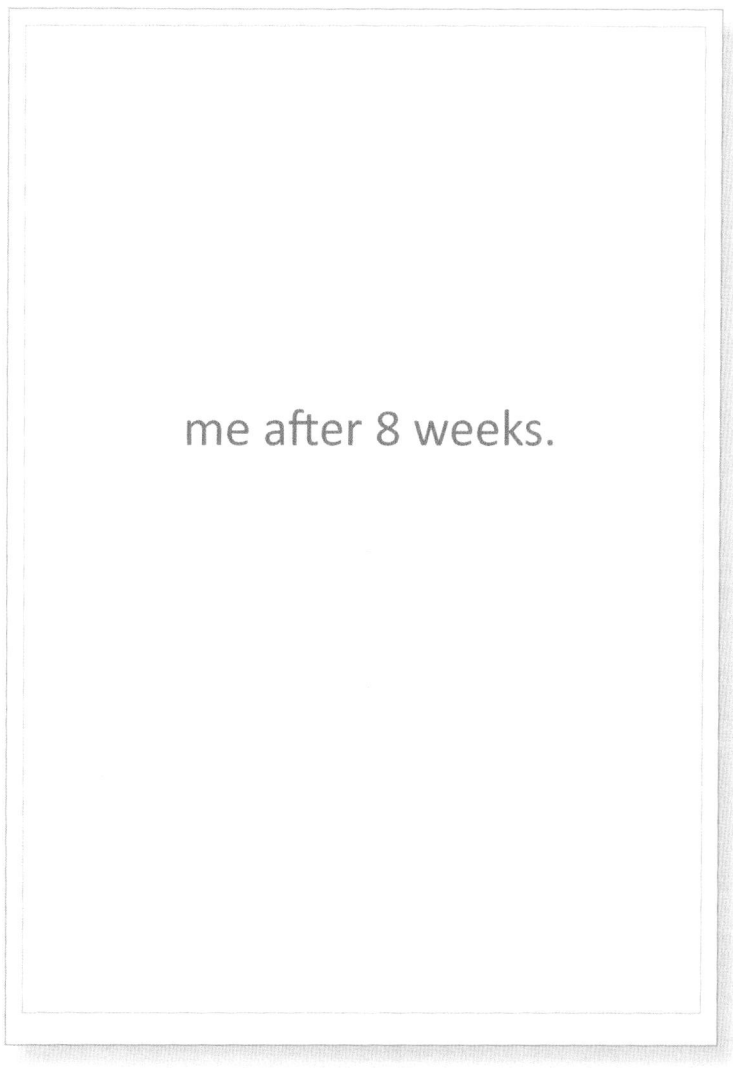

me after 8 weeks.

I lost _____ lbs and _____ inches!

Congratulations!! You knew you could do it.

your act of commitment

I, _____ (your name) will

enlist in *The Original Boot Camp* for the next 8 weeks, from

_____(start date)

to _____(end date, 8 weeks from start).

I want to kick ass. I want to follow this workout and stick with it, and no matter how much my muscles scream at me to stop, I won't. If I have friends come into town, I'm hung over, overworked, sick or tired, I will reschedule my workout but not stop completely, not take more than three days off my workout per month, and I will treat myself like an athlete in training - nutritionally and physically. Because I know I can be 'all that' and its time for me to get a body I am totally proud of once and for all.

Signed _____

Date _____

Witness _____

how to use this book

Each week of *The Original Boot Camp* includes 3 boot camp workouts in addition to 2 to 6 running or power walking sessions of 60 minutes or more. If you prefer to do other forms of cardio, thats fine too - as long as the heart rate is in the right zone.

The boot camp workouts include a 1 mile run, 100 pushups, 100 situps, 10 sets of 30 second sprints and then the strength workout outlined in section 2. This section corresponds to the training weeks - for example, do workout #1, 2 and 3 the first week, and #22, 23, 24 on week 8. The testing day workouts are also included on week 1, 4 and 8.

Most people find it best to make an appointment with themselves and do the same time slot every day - doing the boot camp workout on Monday, Wednesday, Friday morning with an easy cardio session in the evening, and their hardest cardio sessions on Tuesday, Thursday and Saturday. Just be sure to take at least one day off to rest.

The boot camp workouts are done with a time limit, with the goal to do as many as you can in that time frame. You'll watch yourself dramatically improve as the weeks go by.

the basics

Pushups, sit-ups and sprints are the 'basics' of your workout, included before every resistance day. You can modify them to your ability, as long as you still are pushing personal limits. If you're sneeding a few seconds rest every once in a while, you're working at the right level. You'll be surprised how much your 'comfort zone' will change.

With all exercises, make sure you are exhaling with the effort - breathing correctly is super important. So in pushups, for example, you're breathing out as you come up ('blowing yourself up'). Exhale with the effort and try to relax through your muscles, while enjoying the experience!

sprinting

Works: everything!

Goal: Sprint as fast as you can for 30 seconds without stopping, as if your life depended on it. Then stop and rest for up to a minute. Do this 10 times.

SPRINTS: Drive arms forward and propel legs up to chest. Use upper body strength to stabilize torso, calm breathing and move as fast as you can.

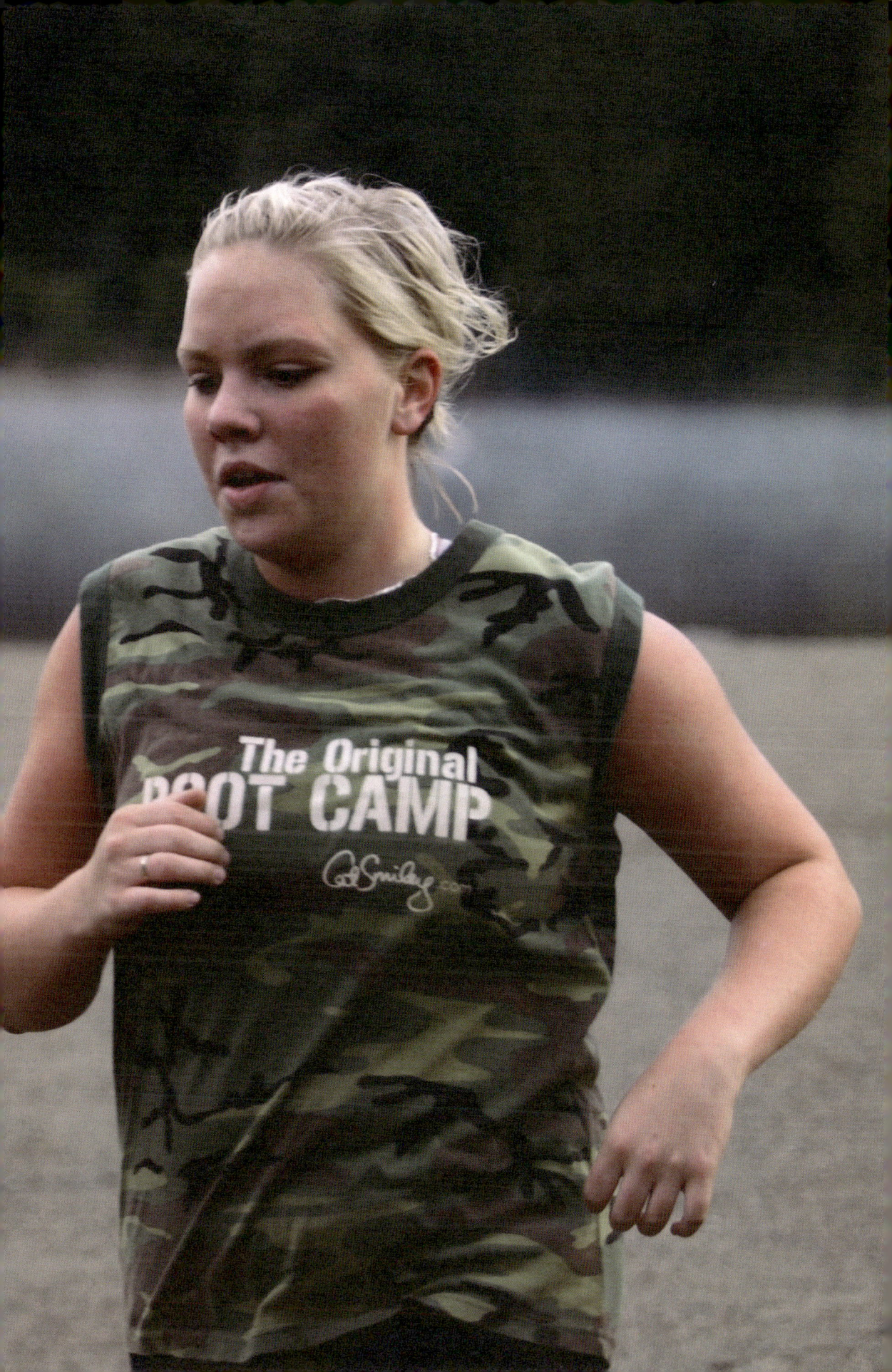

pushups

Works: Chest, arms, core (mid-section) and upper back.

Goal: Keeping your feet and hands your base of support, squeeze the legs and butt, look up slightly and drop your chest below your elbows, relaxing your muscles. Push up quickly and aggressively, to a straight arm position.

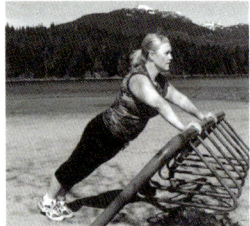 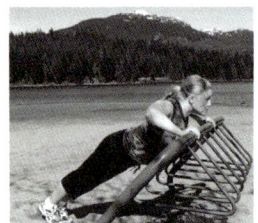

LEVEL 1: Place hands about 3 ft apart, against a wall or platform, such as this bike stand. Dip below elbows, creating a straight line from elbows through collar bone, until you feel a squeeze in your back. Push up, breathing out. Keep your head up, and repeat.

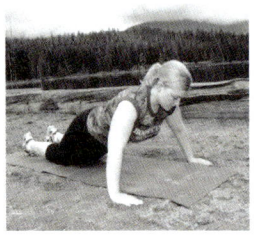 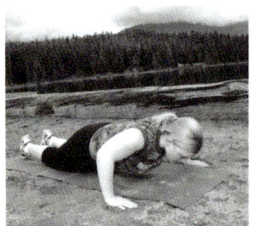

LEVEL 2: Place hands about 3 ft. apart, knees on mat. Dip down below elbows, until you feel a squeeze in your back. Stabilize stomach, and make sure your forearms are vertical at all times. Don't lean back, or stick your butt up!

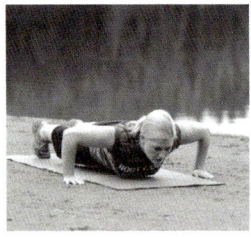 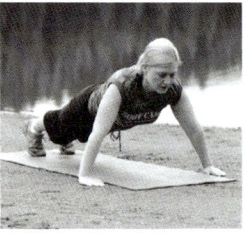

LEVEL 3: Full Pushups! Right on. If you are here, its because you are capable of dipping your chest all the way down, to an inch or two off the ground. Your stomach is tight, with your weight balanced over your hands and feet.

situps

Works: Entire torso

Goal: A full situp is when your feet are flat on the ground (about a foot from your butt), hands are behind the head. Starting position is with the elbows on ground which you will return to after every situp.

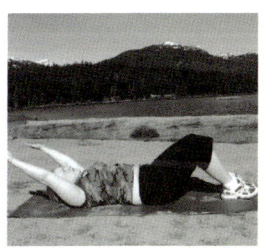 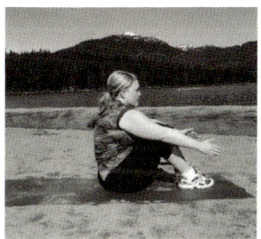

LEVEL 1: Lie on back, arms over head, feet on ground. Throw hands up, finishing in sitting position.

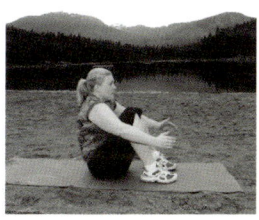 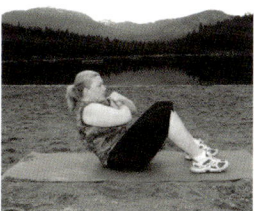

LEVEL 2: Start seated, hands outstretched or across your chest, feet on ground. Recline back to 45 degrees, crunching stomach to return to sitting position.

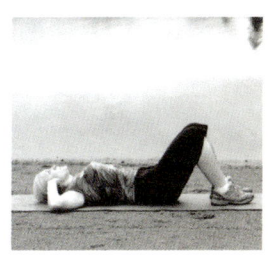 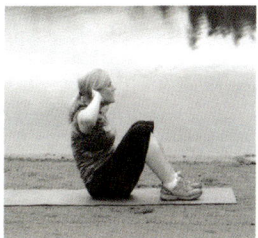

LEVEL 3: Lie on back, hands on ears, feet on ground. Contract abdominals to come up to vertical position, keeping hands on ears.

stretching

Stretching is crucial for injury prevention and to maximize your workout. Never stretch without warming up first. Jump around, go for a quick jog, anything to get some blood flowing. Go through these stretches before each resistance workout, following this order. Hold each lower body stretch for 2-3 minutes, and upper body stretch for 30-60 seconds. Remember to breathe!

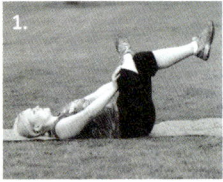

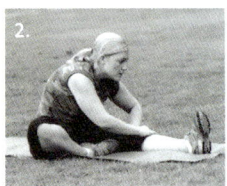

1. HAMSTRINGS AND LOWER BACK: Sit with 1 leg bent and tucked tightly by inner thigh. With a straight back, reach forwards with middle of chest leaning towards middle of knee, toe pointing up. Place pillow on straight leg if you need and push down into it with your elbows.

2. THIGHS: Put legs in a 90°angle, holding ankle of back foot. Lie back and get spine as close to the ground as possible allowing the weight of your legs to stretch thighs. Eventually you'll be able to lie down on the leg.

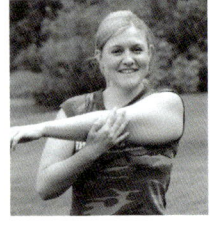

SHOULDER AND NECK: Standing, reach forward with right arm as far as you can while keeping shoulders back. Bring arm across body without raising shoulder. Switch.

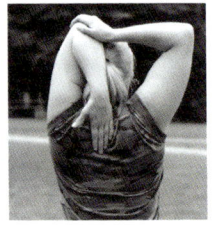

TRICEPS: Standing with perfect posture, place middle finger on the top of spine, keeping head up. Use opposite hand to push elbow back and down.

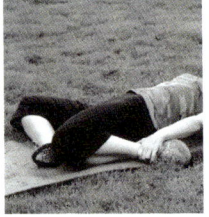

BUTT: Place your right foot on left knee, push right knee back. Keep body straight. Switch.

justine ewart

Exercising regularly has been the best example I can give my daughter. Getting in shape has had positive, positive, positive impact on my ability to be a better Mom. It is so good for her to feed off of me the alertness and happiness that comes with staying in shape. She knows when mommy is going to The Original Boot Camp™.

After about the 21st day since starting The Original Boot Camp™ I noticed a change and felt on my way to a healthy routine. Whistler has great surroundings and easy access to fantastic trails, which makes it easier. If you are finding it hard to get up and go, have a look around and change what is in the way.

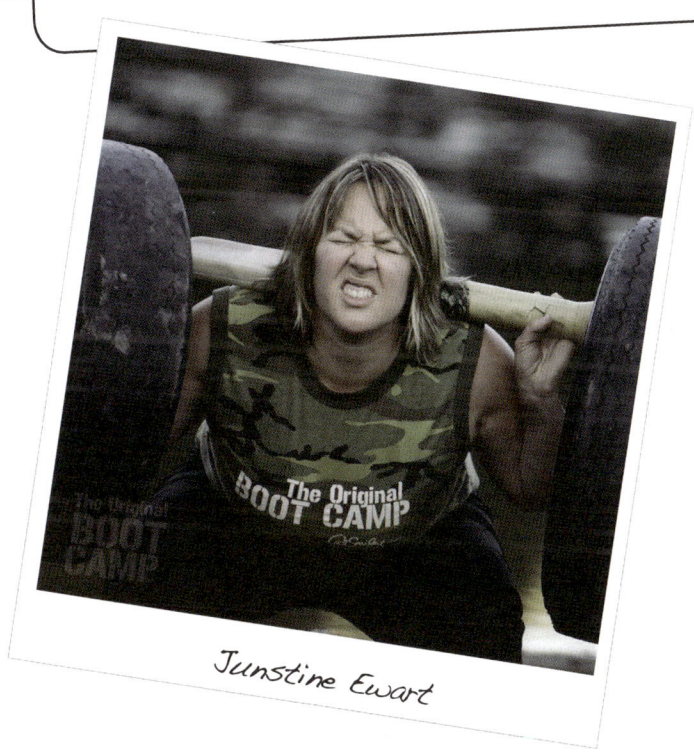

Junstine Ewart

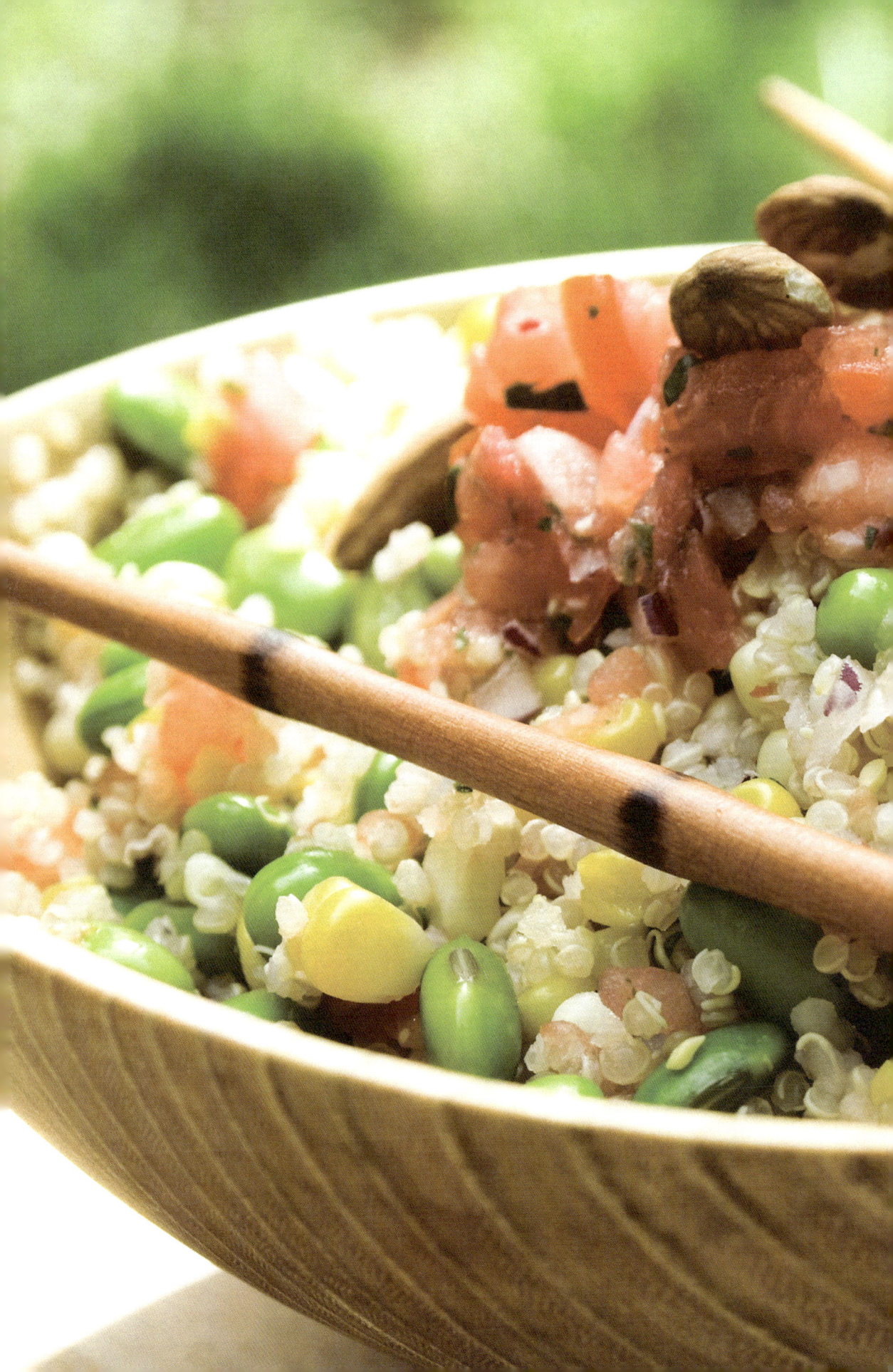

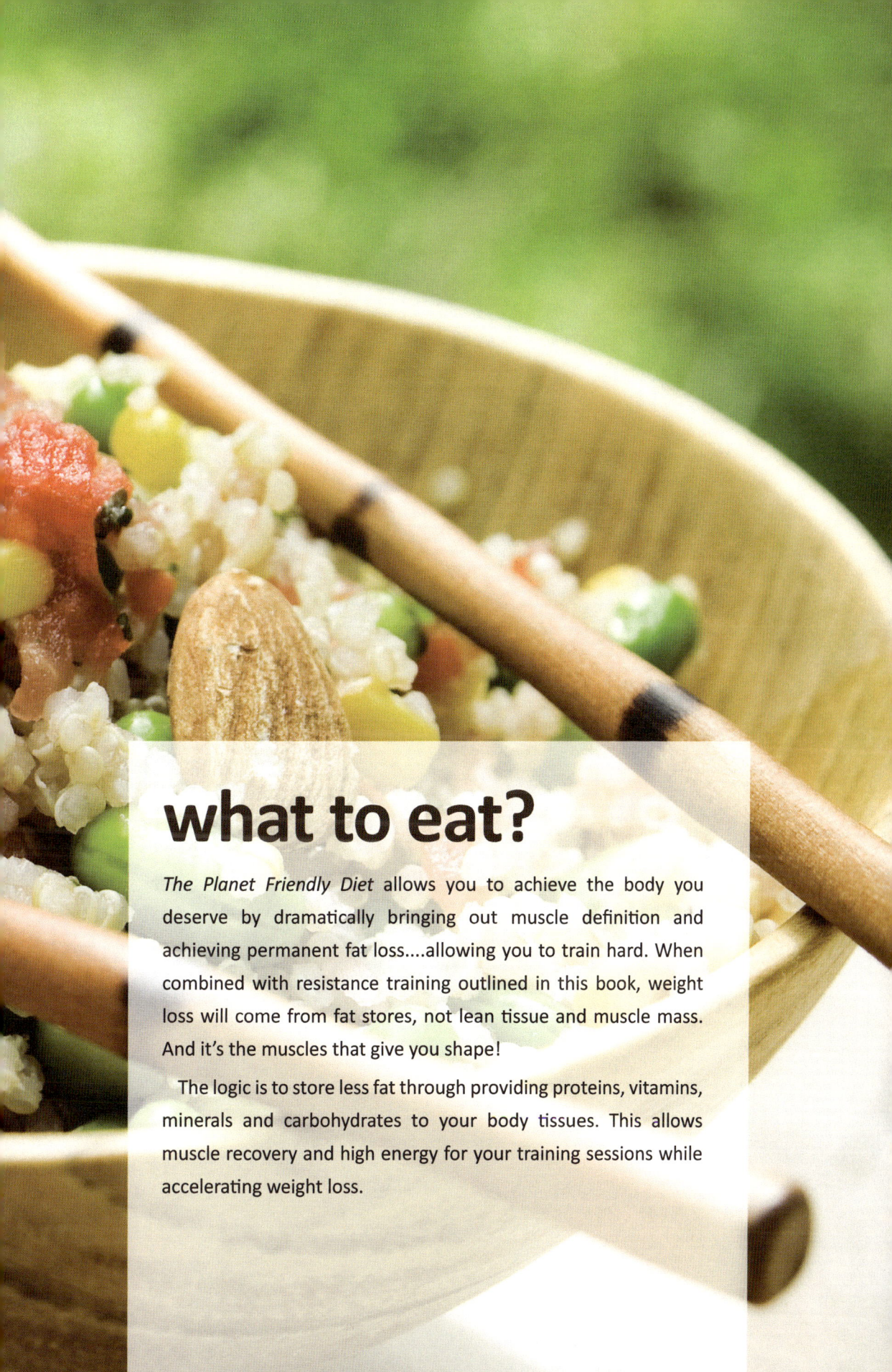

what to eat?

The Planet Friendly Diet allows you to achieve the body you deserve by dramatically bringing out muscle definition and achieving permanent fat loss....allowing you to train hard. When combined with resistance training outlined in this book, weight loss will come from fat stores, not lean tissue and muscle mass. And it's the muscles that give you shape!

The logic is to store less fat through providing proteins, vitamins, minerals and carbohydrates to your body tissues. This allows muscle recovery and high energy for your training sessions while accelerating weight loss.

To maintain weight, but lose fat and gain muscle:

3-4 days per week, on lighter training days, eat 300-500 calories less. Increase your intake for the other 3-4 days by 300-500 calories over five small meals.

To lose weight by losing fat and gaining muscle:

4-5 days per week eat 300-500 calories less than what you would normally eat. Then eat 300-500 calories more than usual, two days per week on heaviest training days.

To gain weight by losing fat and building muscle:

4-5 days per week, increase meal sizes by adding 300-500 calories to total daily consumption (what you would normally eat. Then decrease meal sizes two days per week, eating 300-500 calories less than usual.

"I lost weight and inches, but also became so much stronger and toned. Boot Camp energizes me for the whole day, and makes me conscious about looking after myself, especially my diet. I am now in better shape than I have ever been."   Sonia Mahony, Whistler.

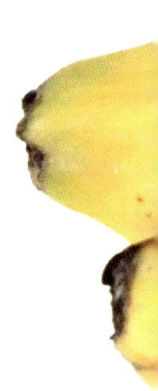

planning your meals

There's nothing worse than being psyched for a good workout, but getting the stitch half way through. These mishaps can be avoided by choosing your foods wisely and also eating them at the right time.

BEFORE	AFTER
Beans	Couscous
Whole wheat bread	Low-fat meats
Granola	Protein shake
Low-fat peanut butter	Banana
Slow cooked oatmeal	Beans
Carrots	Chick peas
Yogurt	Raisin bran
Apple	Sweetcorn
Low-fat milk	Low-fat cheese
Orange juice	Vegetables

SAMPLE WEIGHT LOSS DIET FOR EVENING WORKOUT	
7.30am	2 slices low-carb, high fiber bread, with 2 tsp lite peanut butter. 1 low-fat yogurt. 1 piece fruit.
10.00am	1 cup coffee. 1 piece fruit with cottage cheese.
12.00pm	1 med whole-wheat pita bread with hommus, chickpeas, lettuce, fresh vegetables, cold meat. 2 pieces of fruit.
3.00pm	whey protein shake, with low fat yogurt and banana
5.30pm	WORKOUT
7.30pm	125g lean meat, brown rice, steamed vegetables with thai sauce, 1 tbsp cashew nuts. Berries for desert.

Menu planning can be like stringing together jigsaw pieces, but once you get the hang of it, it'll become second nature. This book has taught you everything you need to know about nutrition, now it's up to you to apply it! Empowered eating is about taking charge of your food choices – having the strength and courage to try new things and make changes. Embrace the challenge like a new chapter in your life, taking time to put fresh, wholesome foods together.

Choose natural ingredients that contrast in colors and textures – foods that look better, taste better too! Mix and match simple foods based on what you are doing on that day. Plan ahead and whenever possible, prep food in advance. Organization will help you stay on track. Think about your meal as a whole dish with a balance of textures, taste and sensations.

Practice mindful eating by being aware of food that trigger certain cravings – for example, salty food always makes people seem to crave sweet so when you're serving salmon, add some vegetables to the plate. Or if you know that you like crisp to follow creamy, find a natural way to include it in your meal. This will save you from looking for something after your meal.

Timing your meals makes a lot of difference in both your athletic performance and weight loss journey. When you exercise on an empty stomach the body looks for muscle tissue to supply energy, instead of stored carbohydrate. It's easier for the body to convert proteins in the muscle tissue into blood glucose when carbohydrates are not found from a recent meal. This deficit triggers a drop in blood-sugar levels though spiking your insulin levels, giving you ox-hunger next time you eat - and revving up the fat-storing enzyme. Aim to eat 6 small meals a day, every couple of hours, so that you never get hungry and overeat. Blend all *3* macronutrients together, based on the information you've learned about in this book. Early morning exercisers should have at least a hundred calories of complex carbohydrate in their system before training – try soy milk latte, a piece of toast, or a rice cracker. Something to wake up your metabolism and give you energy until breakfast.

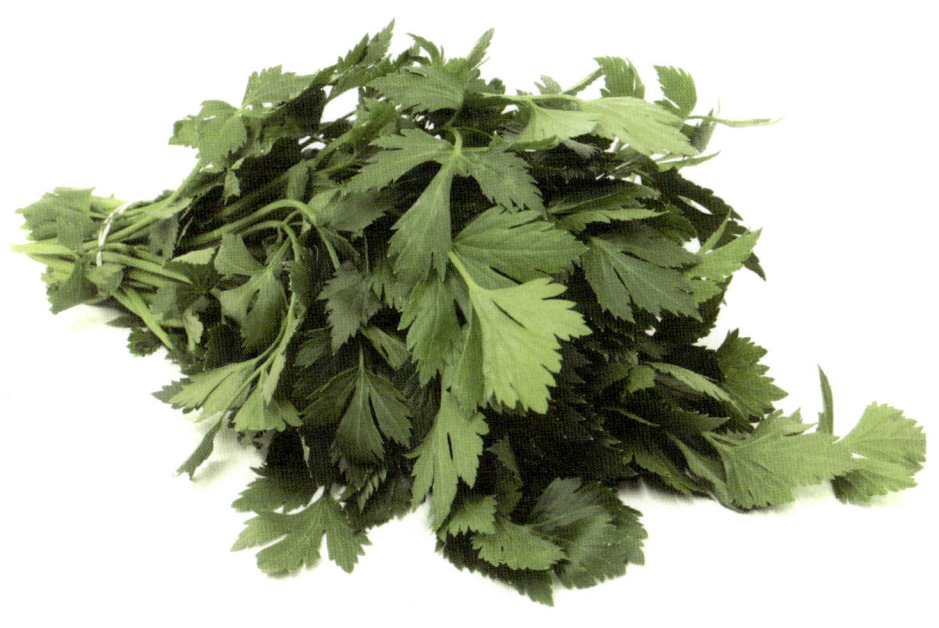

nick davies

I feel much better about myself. I look and feel healthier, sleep better and get more enjoyment out of the physical things I do. I have achieved a net weight reduction of about 40 pounds since starting The Original Boot Camp™, and have lost many inches off of my chest, waist and legs. I have significantly improved my physical condition, and remediation of some old injuries. Since I shed the weight, improved my posture and increased the strength of the muscles that move and carry me around, people react to me entirely differently than the overweight couch potato I used to be. Not only is this apparent on the street or in social settings, but it is also in business meetings.

I asked myself what my true definition of "mentally drained" was and what I could do to address these issues. I have found that participating at The Original Boot Camp™ after a mentally tough day is a good thing. As soon as I start to warm up, I become focused on my exercise and leave everything else behind.

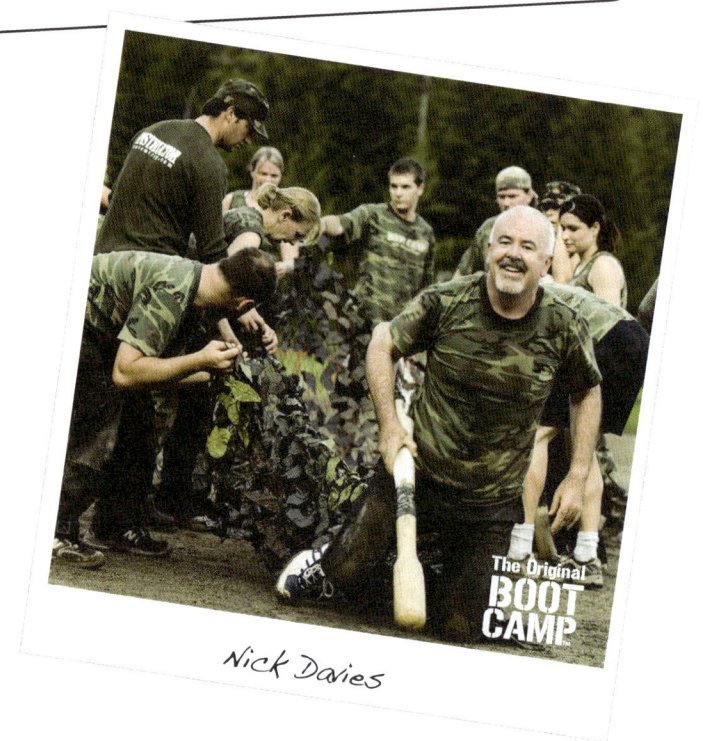

Nick Davies

The fastest fat burning time is 45 minutes after your workout. This is the peak of your digestion cycle where your metabolism enzymes replenish glycogen to the muscles and rebuild protein stores. Eating within this window will allow you to eat more as you'll burn it at a faster rate.

Keep yourself well hydrated throughout the day. Pre-hydration is important - if you wake up in the morning and your urine is dark, get drinking. A good workout will use about 125ml of water every 15 minutes or so (depending on your pre-hydration levels, intensity and climate) therefore keep at least 500ml nearby to replenish hydration.

Breakfast is the time to 'break the fast' of sleeping. When you wake up, you will have gone at least 8 hours without eating. Your body needs nutrition at this point to fuel and energize its vital organs, such as your brain. The nutritional composition of breakfast does not differ greatly from any other meal. A balanced meal should be approximately 20-30% fat, 40-50% carbohydrate and 20-30% protein.

Expand your dietary patterns - eat a whole grain bagel instead of a white bagel, with a whole apple instead of orange juice, use low-fat nut butter or a small handful of trail mix to balance your protein count. Mix your regular *Cheerios* with some old fashioned oatmeal, mixed with real fruit, soymilk or yogurt and almonds. Top your whole-grain English muffin with some low-fat cheese.

Spend money on foods that you enjoy. If you're only going to have 30 grams of cheese with tonight's meal, why buy $6 cheddar? Splurge out! Buy that $12 cheese and savour it. Enjoy a little bit and be satisfied.

Think quality over quantity: often we eat too much because we're looking for satisfaction in taste sensation. You don't have to eat a lot of food to make it work for you - you just have to make the right choices. Breakfast needs to be as balanced nutritionally as any other meal, so get with the modern way of eating and start your day with energy!

There are thousands of delicious natural foods to choose from and this book shows you how easy it is to eat properly. Turn back the clock and rekindle your appreciation of taste — notice if it's sweet, savoury, sour or spicy. Become a food combining super star by learning how to plate dishes beautifully, whether the ingredients are grilled, roasted, simmered, boiled or steamed. Mix up your serving style using high fiber options — a bed of raw spinach, or a red pepper stuffed with brown rice.

There are always going to be a bumper crop of vegetables available at your local farmers market, packed full of fiber, nutrients and flavour. Learn to use them as the main feature in your recipe, not just as an accompaniment. Soups, hot pots, casseroles....use their vibrant colors to elevate your mood and energy! Cool down dishes with soy yogurt instead of cream or butter.

Yogurt can be used as a healthy substitute in pretty much anything. Eat foods raw as much as possible, to get the full nutritional benefits. Drink water throughout the day, and go easy on all other beverages. Plan your shopping ahead of time so that you can bring a reusable bag with you, which saves plastic. Grow your own herbs and spices…. even better, plant a vegetable garden.

> Go global in your food inspiration – draw from cultures around the world to combine pulses, whole wheat flour, fruit and vegetables.

Spare some thought for the communities outside your home town and the labour it took to bring tonight's meal to your dinner table. For products you can't source locally, buy *Fair Trade*. This ensures that the farmer is paid fairly, which means their employees are more likely to be treated fairly, contributing to the planet friendly goal of your diet.

Experiment with different flavour variations of herbs and spices. There are so many combinations to stumble upon. Memorize the foods that are high fiber and include them in at least one dish per day. Learn the tricks of the trade, like using nuts and seeds to keep the meal crunchy and crispy, without the use of processed crackers.

Awesomeness starts in the kitchen – **kick start your change** and make it a habit. Life is best served low fat and high energy!

how to measure

date_____

Chest: Over center, arms up

Waist: Over belly button

Hips: Over widest part

Thigh: Under clenched fist, with arm straight against leg

For accurancy, have the same friend measure you each time.

your measurements

	WEEK 1	WEEK 4	WEEK 8
CHEST			
WAIST			
HIPS			
THIGH			

Calculate your total shrinkage over the past 8 weeks. Double the inches lost in your thighs - you have 2 legs!		
	WEEK 4	WEEK 8 (TOTAL)
WEIGHT LOST		
INCHES LOST		

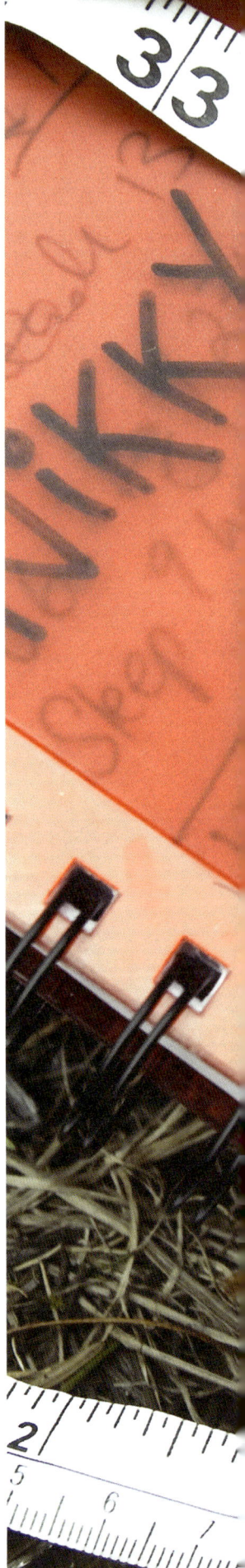

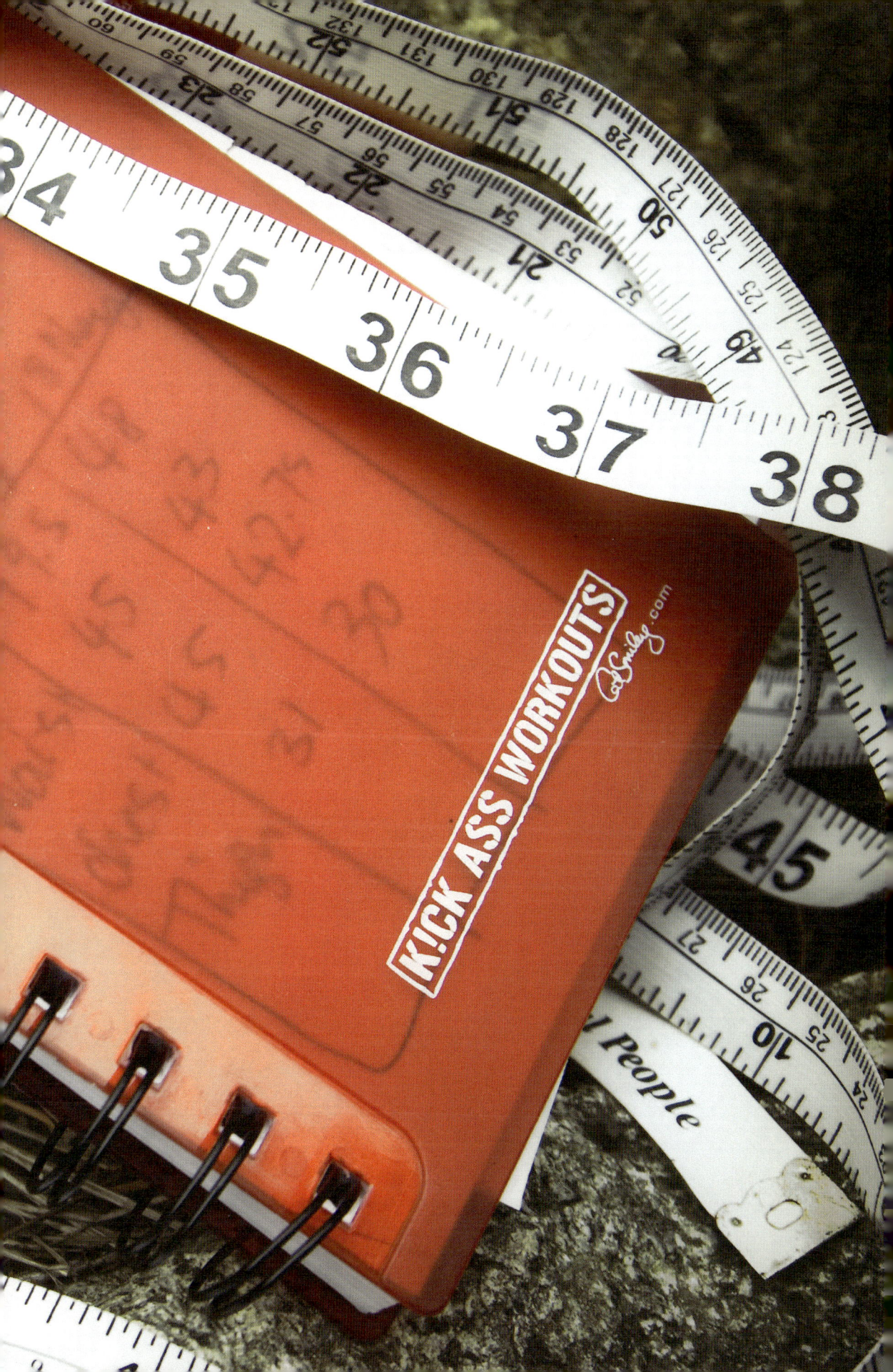

how to test

Only the exercises performed with perfect form count - as demonstrated on the next page.

RUN	Time how long it takes, running your heart out for 1 mile (1.6kms)
MAX PUSHUPS	Be honest!
TRICEP DIPS	As many as you can in 2 minutes.
MAX SITUPS	Many recruits are surprised to learn they can't do any.
PLANK	Hold a plank until you collapse.

EXERCISE	WEEK 1	WEEK 4	WEEK 8	GOALS
RUN 1.6km/1mile				
PUSHUPS total without stopping				
TRICEP DIPS total in 2 minutes				
SITUPS total without stopping				
PLANK Maximum				

testing exercises

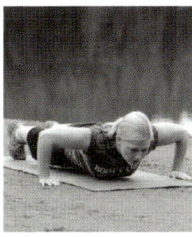 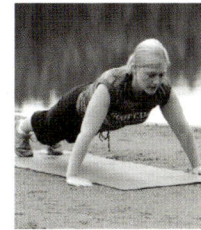

PUSH UP: Place hands about three feet apart, horizontal to your collar bone (elbows up). Dip chest all the way down, to an inch or two off the ground, keeping back completely straight. Your stomach is stable, your weight balanced over your hands and feet.

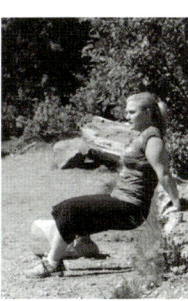 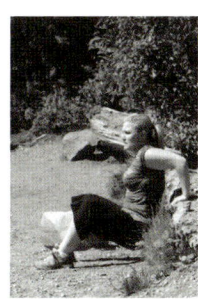

TRICEPS DIP: Sit down and place hands beside your butt, elbows directly behind you. Feet are firmly placed on the ground, knees bent and toes relaxed. Dip down so that the backs of your arms are horizontal to the ground, forearms vertical. Breathe out as you come up.

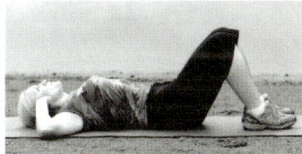 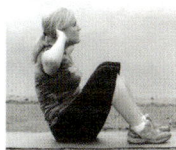

SIT UP: Lie on back, hands on ears feet firmly planted on the ground. Use your stomach strength to come up to sitting position. Hands stay on ears, feet stay on the ground.

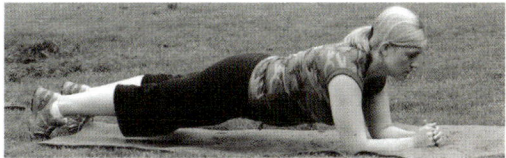

PLANK: Place elbows on the ground directly under armpits (hands in prayer position) with back and legs perfectly straight. Weight is on your toes and elbows. Imagine you are a plank of wood - dead straight!

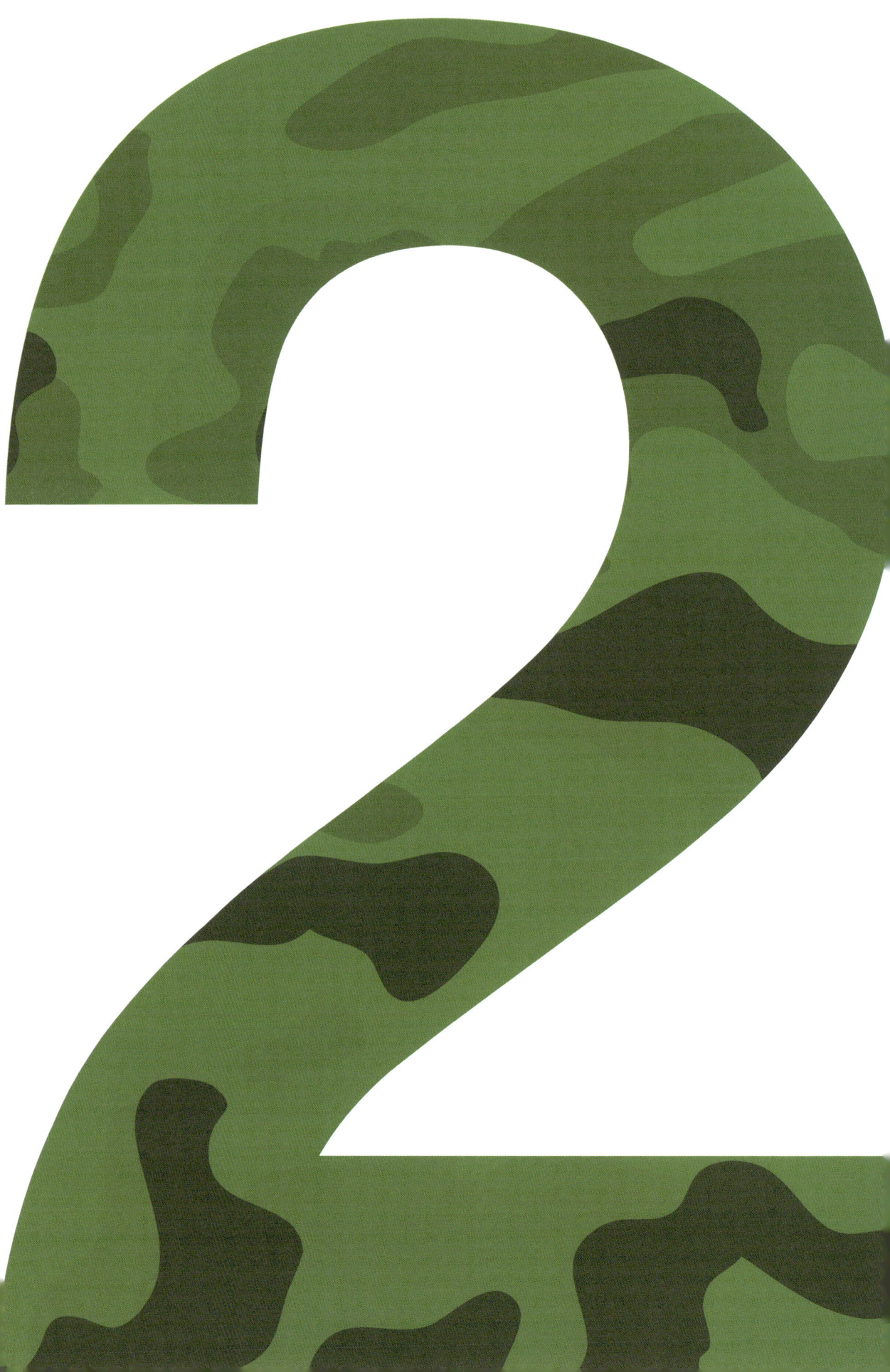

24 kick ass workouts

workout 1

1 mile run + basics + sprints + core = kick ass workout

Facing your testing results yesterday might have been an eye-opener. But it doesn't matter where you are now, its where you are in eight weeks that counts.

EXERCISE	YOUR GOAL	TIME LIMIT	How many did you do?
Alternate between exercises 1 and 2.			
1. ALTERNATING TOE TOUCH	2 x 25 on each side	6 mins	
2. PLANK	2 x 30 secs	2 min	
Alternate between exercises 3 and 4.			
3. SUPERMAN	2 x 25	2 min	
4. FLUTTER KICK	2 x 50 on each side	5 mins	

 Fitness goes beyond the physical.
Ever noticed how much easier it is to train when you have a happy home?

your exercises today

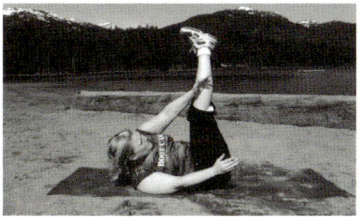 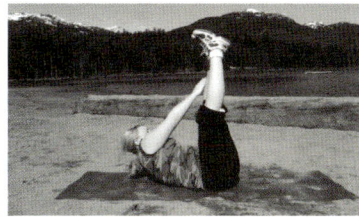

1. ALTERNATING TOE TOUCH: Lie on your back, feet directly up in the air. Reach across body and chop ankles. You should feel the burn in your sides. If this hurts your neck, put your hands behind your head and bend the knees.

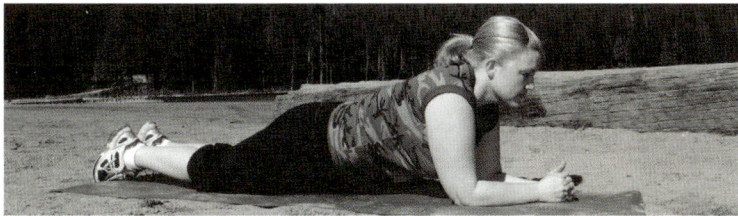

2. PLANK: Place elbows on the ground directly under armpits (hands in prayer position) with back and legs perfectly straight. Weight is on your toes and elbows. This is the modified version shown - if you feel up to it, lift knees off the ground.

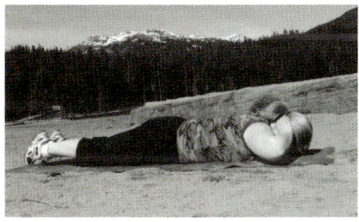 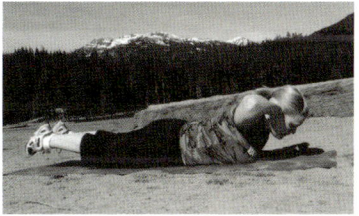

3. SUPERMAN: Lie on stomach, arms outstretched in flying position or under your chin, legs straight and off the ground. Lift up chest to maximum extension and pulse up and down about 3 inches.

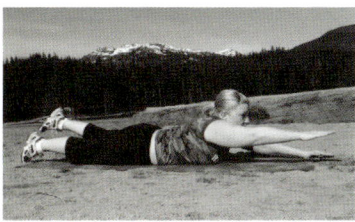 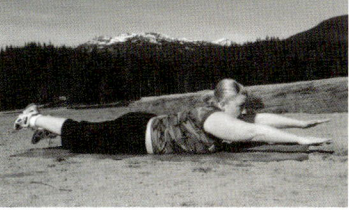

4. FLUTTER KICK: Lie on stomach, lift right arm up and left leg up at the same time, keeping arms and legs off the ground. Switch. Remember to breathe! Keep head down if this aggravates your neck.

workout 2 lower

1 mile run + basics + sprints + lower = kick ass workout

You'll wake up sore this morning (mostly in your chest and arms)
so really stretch well. It's great you're doing this for yourself.
Taking care of number one!

EXERCISE	YOUR GOAL	TIME LIMIT	How many did you do?
Alternate between exercises 1 and 2.			
1. LUNGE WALKS	4 x 10	8 mins	
2. JUMP SQUATS	4 x 10	2 mins	
Alternate between exercises 3 and 4.			
3. SIDE SQUAT on log	3 x 6 on each side	5 mins	
4. INDIVIDUAL LUNGE	3 x 6 on each side	5 mins	

*Hungry? Blame it on science! Increased appetite in fall is nature's way of
fattening us up for winter. Fight it by boosting your metabolism – get outside,
run around, get active. It's a great day out there*

your exercises today

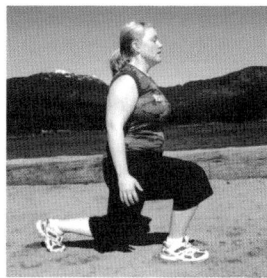 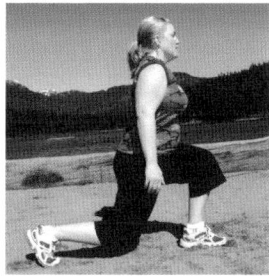

LUNGE WALKS: Builds the endurance in your legs. Take a big step forward, and lower yourself down so that your front leg is horizontal. Create a square and make sure the knees never go over your toes. Keep your torso straight.

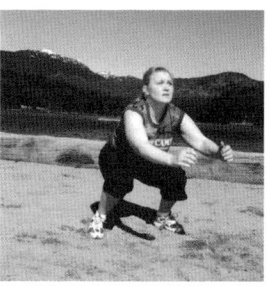 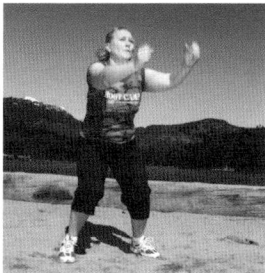

JUMP SQUATS: this explosive work will make sure you don't get bulky after those lunge walks! Keep your feet wide, torso strong, head up, stick your butt out and make sure the knees never go over your toes. Look up.

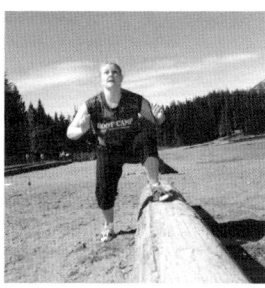 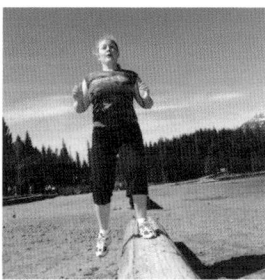 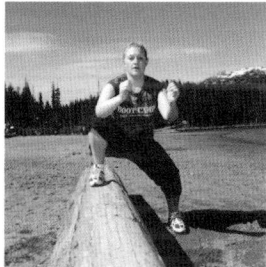

SIDE SQUAT ON LOG: Inner thighs baby, all the way. Stick your butt right out and lower yourself down keeping the front knee over your foot. Explode up and over the log, but be careful to keep your balance. This exercise can also be done on the ground.

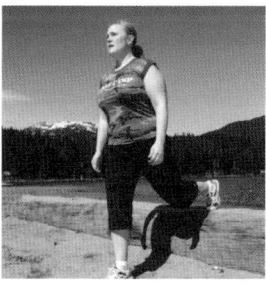 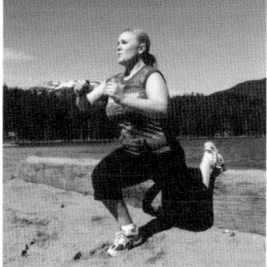

INDIVIDUAL LUNGE: Place back foot on log, (either toes or front of foot, depending on preference) and sink down so your front leg is horizontal. Again, don't let the knee go over your toes. Come up using strength from the leg on the log. You'll also feel a stretch/burn in the back of the other leg.

workout 3 upper

1 mile run + basics + sprints + upper = kick ass workout

Almost through the first week! Did you know that the arms usually tone up faster than any other body part?

Stick with it and you'll see results in three weeks!

EXERCISE	YOUR GOAL	TIME LIMIT	How many did you do?
Alternate between exercises 1 and 2.			
1.OVERHEAD SHOULDER RAISE	2 x 12 each side	6 mins	
2. INDIVIDUAL SHOULDER RAISE	2 x 12 each side	4 mins	
Alternate between exercises 3 and 4.			
3. BICEP CURL	2 x 12 each side	4 mins	
4. TRICEP DIP	2 x 12	4 mins	

 Time-crunched training is sometimes the best way to go. Keep the heart rate elevated by super setting opposite muscle groups – no rest. Just power through!

your exercises today

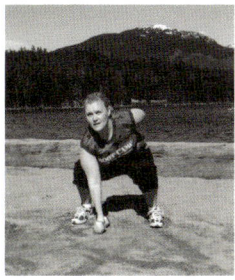 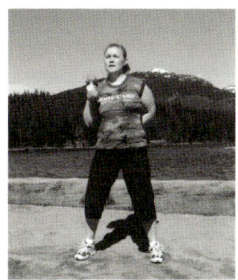 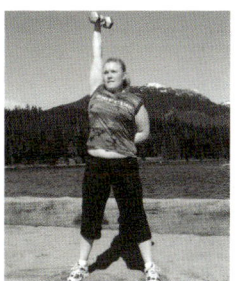

OVERHEAD SHOULDER RAISE: Start in squat position, left hand in the small of lower back, torso strong, head and chest up. Lift quickly up to arm pit, above your head, back to armpit, back to the ground and repeat.

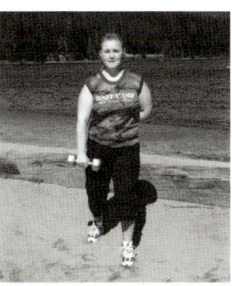 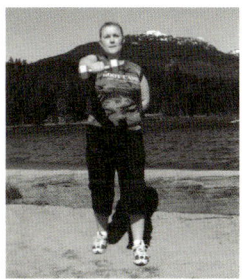

INDIVIDUAL SHOULDER RAISE: Stand with right leg forward in athletic position, lifting left arm up to shoulder height. Bend arm slightly, and feel your shoulder moving and nothing else. Keep torso still, bend knees slightly.

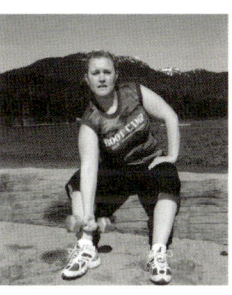 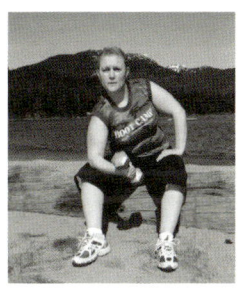 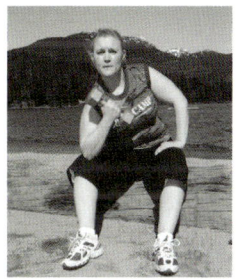

BICEP CURL: Sit down with calf on an angle, elbow in the groove of your knee. Curl up on an angle, into your arm pit. Twist your wrist at the top, keeping your grip relaxed.

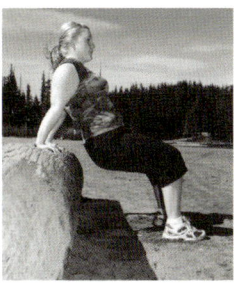 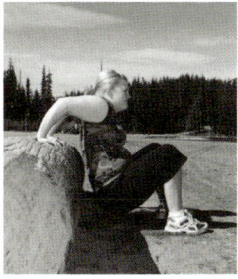

TRICEP DIP: Sit down and place hands beside your butt, elbows directly behind you, fingers facing forward. Feet are firmly placed on the ground, knees bent and toes relaxed. Dip down so that the backs of your arms are horizontal to the ground, forearms vertical. Breathe out as you come up.

workout 4 core

1 mile run + basics + sprints + core = kick ass workout

It's normal to have a tough time on Monday's getting back into the swing of things, but LETS GO!!!!!!!!! Come on! Yes you!!!!!!!!!

EXERCISE	YOUR GOAL	TIME LIMIT	How many did you do?
Alternate between exercises 1 and 2.			
1. SLOW SWIM	3 x 15	2 mins	
2. SUPERMAN	3 x 20	2 mins	
Alternate between exercises 3 and 4.			
3. BOMBER CRUNCH	3 x 12	8 mins	
4. FLUTTER CRUNCH	3 x 12	5 mins	

When you start winning the weight loss game, compliments will happen and it can be challenging to accept them gracefully (we've been taught our whole lives to be humble). Take a deep breath, smile and find your self-esteem. Enjoy the attention – you deserve it!

your exercises today

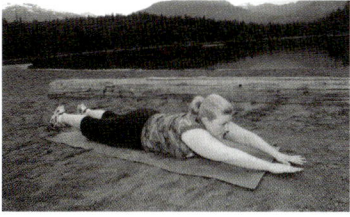 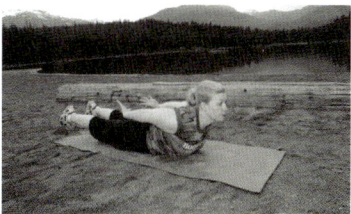

SLOW SWIM: Lie on stomach, hands in front of you and feet off the ground. Squeeze arms back slowly in a breast stroke swimming movement and squeeze shoulder blades together, holding until it hurts!

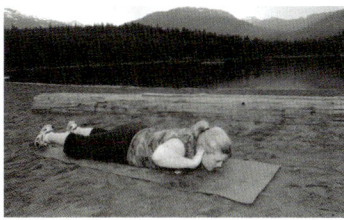 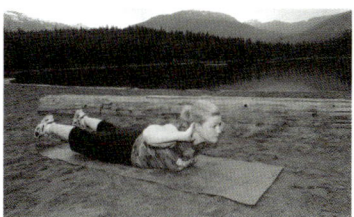

SUPERMAN: Lie on stomach, arms outstretched in flying position or under your chin, legs straight and off the ground. Lift up chest to maximum extension and pulse up and down about 3 inches.

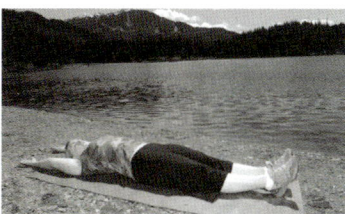 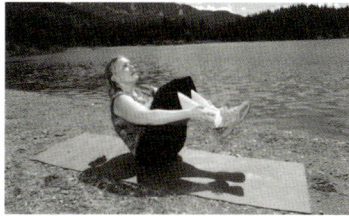

BOMBER CRUNCH: Lie on back, arms straight and outstretched over the head, legs on the ground. Throw arms up explosively and bend knees in a cannon ball, touching hands to ankles. Collapse back to starting position and do it all again.

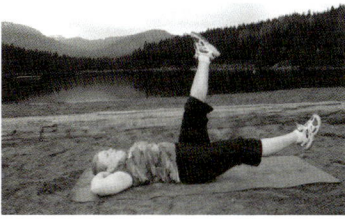 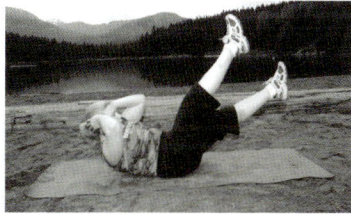

FLUTTER CRUNCH: Lie on back, hands comfortably behind head, legs up in the air. Alternate legs back and forth, only going down as far as you can keep your lower back on the ground. Don't let hip flexors click. Crunch upwards every time the right leg comes up (not side to side) bringing shoulders off the ground.

workout 5 lower

1 mile run + basics + sprints + lower = kick ass workout

The hardest thing today will be the sprints and lunge walks. And the knee ups. Okay, everything. But you can do it - it's one hour of your life.

EXERCISE	YOUR GOAL	TIME LIMIT	How many did you do?
Alternate between exercises 1 and 2.			
1. LUNGE WALK	5 x 10	9 mins	
2. JUMP SQUATS	5 x 10	4 mins	
Alternate between exercises 3 and 4.			
3. KNEE UPS	3 x 6 each side	8 mins	
4. SIDE SQUAT on log	3 x 6 each side	5 mins	

 Dogs make the best trainers! The most enthusiastic running partners, always ready for the trails. Whether you're slow, fast, sad or happy, dogs are just thrilled to be out with you. We should all be so excited about exercising!

your exercises today

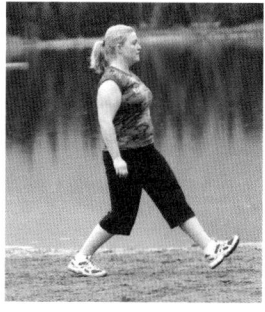 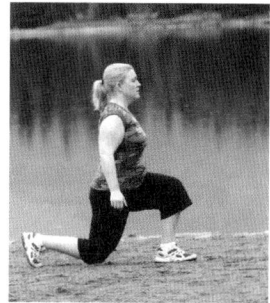

LUNGE WALKS: Take a big step forward, and lower yourself down so that your front leg is horizontal. Create a square and make sure the knees never go over your toes. Look up.

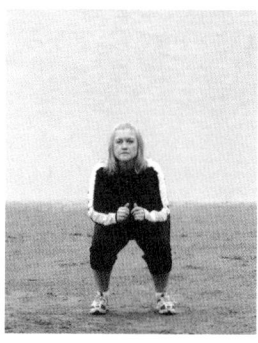 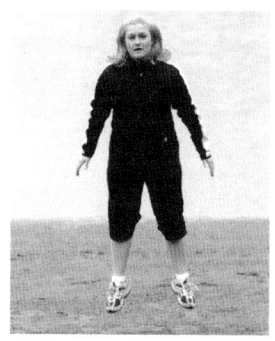

JUMP SQUATS: Keep your feet wide, torso strong, head up, and make sure the knees never go over your toes.

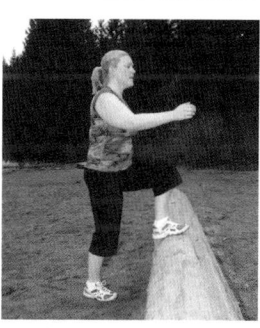 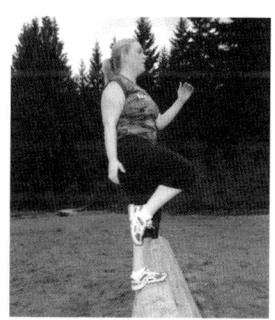

KNEE UPS: Plant right foot firmly on log or bench. Drive left leg up to chest explosively, tap down on the ground and drive it right back up. Use your arms to balance yourself. This might make you feel light headed.

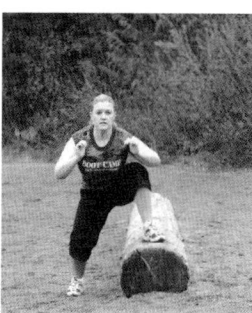 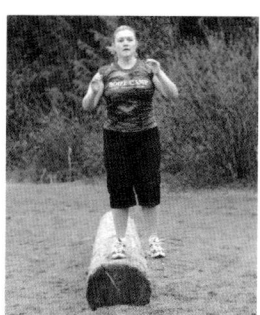 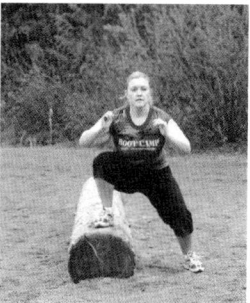

SIDE LUNGE: Place right foot on log or bench, sticking butt out in squat position. Push off right foot to get over the log, and sink down into a squat position on the other side of the log. Repeat. Look up, and place your foot carefully.

workout 6 upper

1 mile run + basics + sprints + upper = kick ass workout

Take your time to do the exercise correctly. Even if the rep count is high, rushing through exercises only increases the risk of injury.

Just do the best you can.

EXERCISE	YOUR GOAL	TIME LIMIT	How many did you do?
Alternate between exercises 1 and 2.			
1. SHOULDER PRESS	3 x 10	3 mins	
2. LATERAL RAISE	3 x 10	2 mins	
Alternate between exercises 3 and 4.			
3. TRICEP PRESS	3 x 15	3 mins	
4. BICEP CURL	3 x 15 each side	6 mins	

Just because you're sweating, doesn't mean you are working in the right zone. Sweat is your body's way to regulate temperature. The heart has to work in the target zone to burn fat.

your exercises today

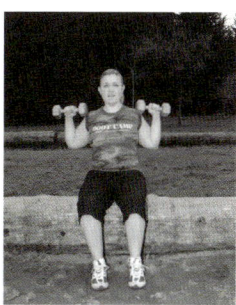 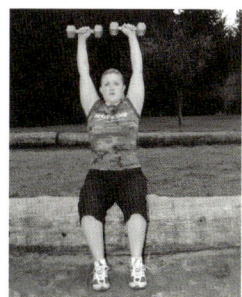

SHOULDER PRESS: Sit with torso straight (without arching your back) and weights balanced at shoulder height. Push up until arms are straight, twisting wrists slightly at the top point. Bring down, squeezing shoulder blades - elbows as low down your sides as possible. Push back up using your shoulder strength.

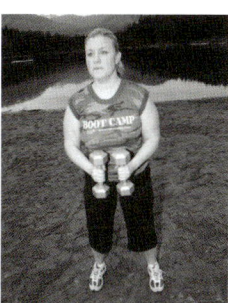 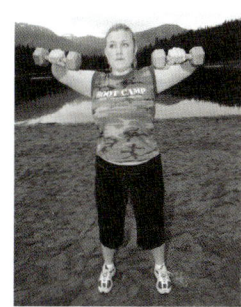

LATERAL RAISE: Standing in athletic position, ankles, knees and hips flexed. Push off toes and raise arms to the side, leading with your elbows. Do not bring the hands past your elbows. Squeeze shoulder blades as you come up, and squeeze the chest as you come down.

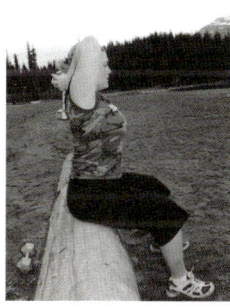 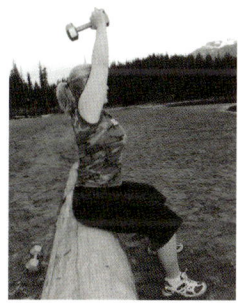

TRICEP PRESS: Sit down, feet firmly planted on the ground, torso slightly forwards. Start with weight touching the back of your spine, elbows over your ears. Push up weight until arms are straight. Make sure you always keep elbows close to head.

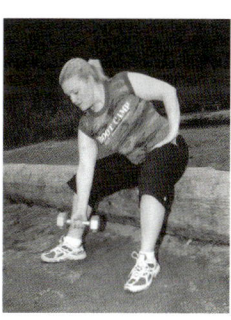 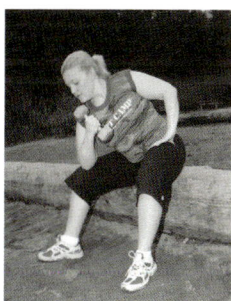

BICEP CURL: Sit with feet apart, legs on an angle. The calf will support your curl. Put elbow is in the groove of your knee and curl up into your arm pit. Twist your wrist at the top. Keep grip relaxed.

workout 7 core

1 mile run + basics + sprints + core = kick ass workout

Shake up your run on occasion with a different route.

You don't need to test yourself every workout - once a week is plenty.

EXERCISE	YOUR GOAL	TIME LIMIT	How many did you do?
Alternate between exercises 1 and 2.			
1. INDIVIDUAL LEG DROPS	3 x 10 each side	6 mins	
2. BOMBER CRUNCH	3 x 15	8 mins	
Alternate between exercises 3 and 4.			
3. SUPERMAN	3 x 15	2 mins	
4. FLUTTER KICK	3 x 30	2 mins	

 Eat mushrooms! This super-food contains the same savoury flavouring (umami) found in fattening foods....and it breaks down carbs. So next time you're craving French fries, cook up some mushrooms instead!

your exercises today

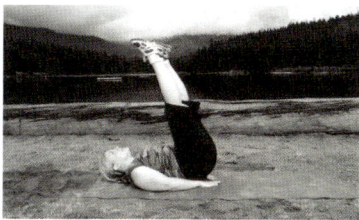 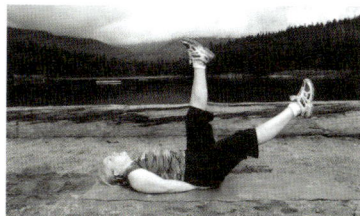

INDIVIDUAL LEG DROP: Lie on back, legs vertical and hands under your butt. Alternate legs back and forth, only going down as far as you can keep your lower back on the ground.

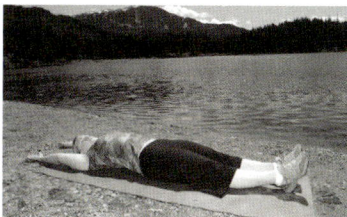 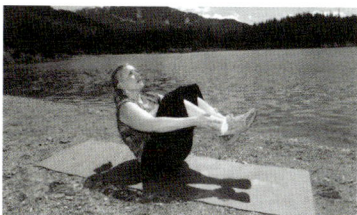

BOMBER CRUNCH: Lie on back, arms straight and outstretched over the head, legs on the ground. Throw arms up explosively and bend knees in a cannon ball, touching hands to ankles. Collapse back to starting position and do it all again.

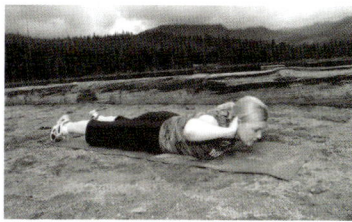 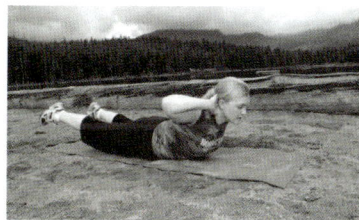

SUPERMAN: Lie on stomach, arms outstretched in flying position or under your chin, legs straight and off the ground. Lift up chest to maximum extension and pulse up and down 3 inches.

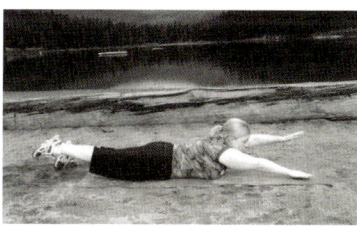 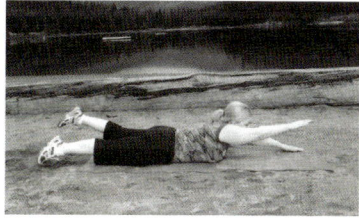

FLUTTER KICK: Lie on stomach, lift right arm up and left leg up at the same time, keeping left arm and right leg off the ground. Switch. Remember to breathe! Keep head down if this aggravates your neck. Don't let hands or feet touch the ground.

workout 8 lower

1 mile run + basics + sprints + lower = kick ass workout

Pay close attention to your technique - especially when you get tired.

The knee ups make recruits feel clumsy. Push yourself at your own pace.

EXERCISE	YOUR GOAL	TIME LIMIT	How many did you do?
Alternate between exercises 1 and 2.			
1. LUNGE WALKS	6 x 10	10 mins	
2. JUMP SQUATS	6 x 10	4 mins	
Alternate between exercises 3 and 4.			
3. INDIVIDUAL LUNGE	3 x 12 each side	9 mins	
4. KNEE UPS	3 x 12 each side	10 mins	

If beauty is in the eye of the beholder, why not make ourselves the 'beholder'?
Free yourself from what others think! It's what you think that counts.

your exercises today

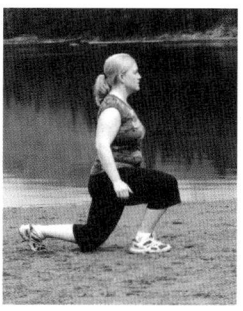 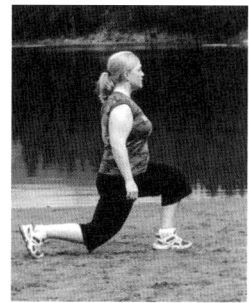

LUNGE WALKS: Take a big step forward, and lower yourself down so that your front leg is horizontal. Create a square and make sure the knees never go over your toes.

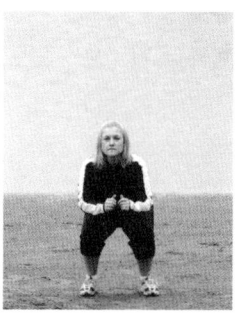 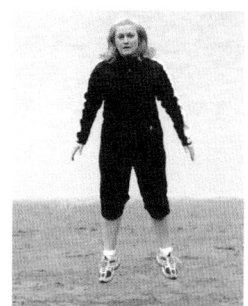

JUMP SQUATS: Keep your feet wide, torso strong, head up, and with the knees never going over your toes in the squat position. Stick your butt out and jump up, fully extended.

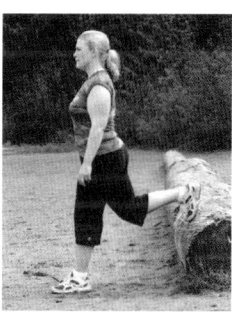 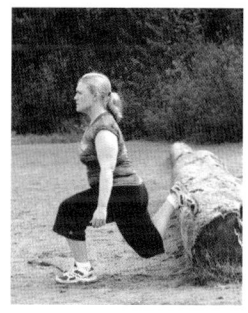

INDIVIDUAL LUNGE: Place back foot on log, and sink down so your front leg is horizontal. Come up using strength from the leg on the log. You'll also feel a stretch/burn in the back of the other leg.

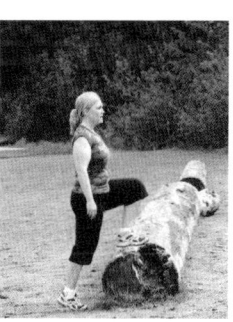 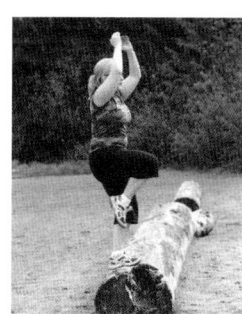

KNEE UPS: Plant right foot firmly on log or bench. Drive left leg up to chest explosively, tap down on the ground and drive it right back up. Use your arms however you like to balance yourself.

workout 10 upper

1 mile run + basics + sprints + upper = kick ass workout

And you thought you couldn't do it. Good job!

No-one said it would be easy.

EXERCISE	YOUR GOAL	TIME LIMIT	How many did you do?
Alternate between exercises 1 and 2.			
1. INDIVIDUAL SHOULDER RAISE	3 x 15 each side	6 mins	
2. PUNCH THRU	3 x 15 each side	4 mins	
Alternate between exercises 3 and 4.			
3. TRICEP PRESS	3 x 15	3 mins	
4. BICEP CURL	3 x 15 each side	6 mins	

 Today is the day to face whatever fear it is that's holding you back from being the athlete you're capable of bring. Open yourself to change and go get the life you want! It may be easier than you think.

your exercises today

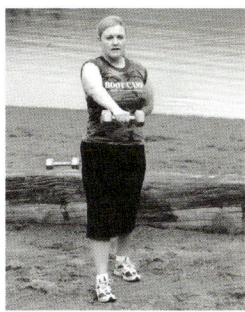 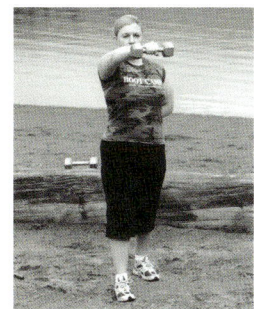

INDIVIDUAL SHOULDER RAISE: Stand with right leg forward in athletic position, lifting left arm up to shoulder height. Bend arm - feel your shoulder moving and nothing else. Keep torso still, bend knees slightly.

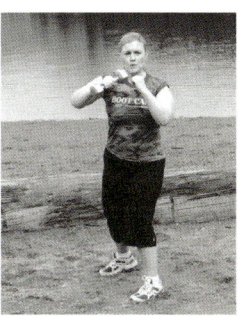 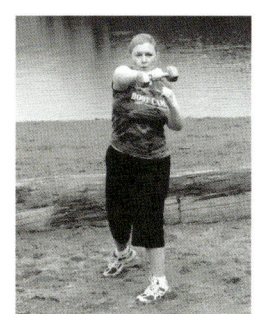

PUNCH THRU: Stand with left leg forward (knee bent) and right hand holding weight close to your face. Keeping elbow close to body, punch out aggressively, twisting wrist at the impact point (the end). Snap back weight to your face. Don't let your hands drop! Give 'er!

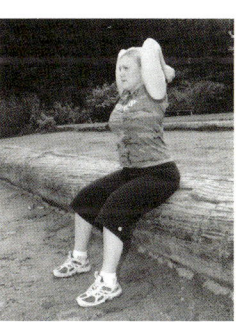 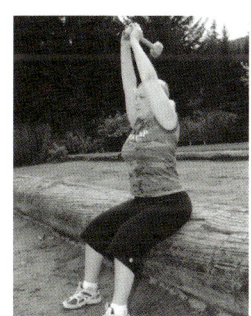

TRICEP PRESS: Sit down, feet firmly planted, torso slightly forwards. Start with weight touching the back of your spine, elbows over your ears. Push up the weight until arms are straight. Make sure you always keep elbows close to head.

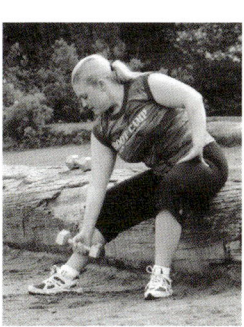 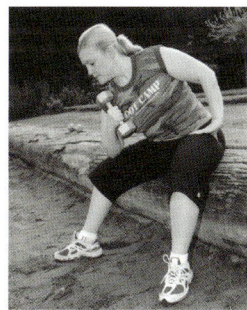

BICEPS CURL: Sitting with calf angled and elbow in the groove of your knee. Curl up on an angle, into your arm pit. Twist your wrist at the top. Don't collapse torso.

workout 11 core

1 mile run + basics + sprints + core = kick ass workout

Every exercise can be easy or excruciatingly hard. For example, the slow swim - the easy version is fast, but that's not our goal. Push yourself!

EXERCISE	YOUR GOAL	TIME LIMIT	How many did you do?
Alternate between exercises 1 and 2.			
1. BOMBER CRUNCHES	3 x 15	8 mins	
2. V-UPS	3 x 10	8 mins	
Alternate between exercises 3 and 4.			
3. SLOW SWIM	3 x 15	2 mins	
4. PLANK	3 x 1 min	3 mins	

 No-one can lead, motivate or inspire you to shape up unless you have made the decision to do so. Take the first step to a fitter you – you can do this!

your exercises today

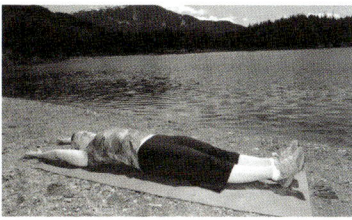 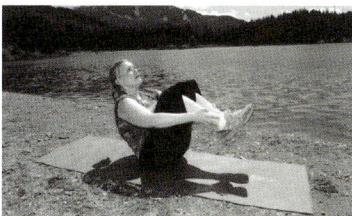

BOMBER CRUNCH: Lie on back, arms straight and outstretched over the head, legs on the ground. Throw arms up explosively and bend knees in a cannon ball, touching hands to ankles. Collapse back to starting position and do it all again. And again.

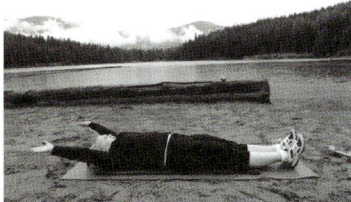 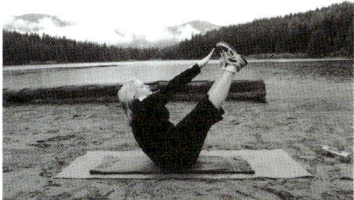

V-UPS: Exactly the same as the bomber crunch, except with straight legs - and even harder! Throw arms up agressively so the torso comes up quicker than the legs. Aim to touch toes, like a divers pike, raise chest high & look up!

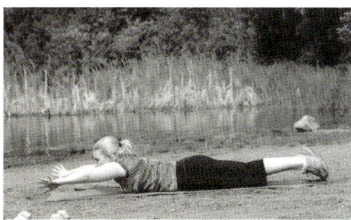 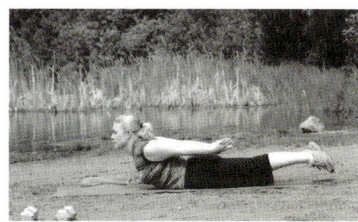

SLOW SWIM: Lie on stomach, hands in front of you and feet off the ground. Squeeze arms back slowly in a breast stroke swimming movement and squeeze shoulder blades together, holding until it hurts! Lift feet off ground when hands come back.

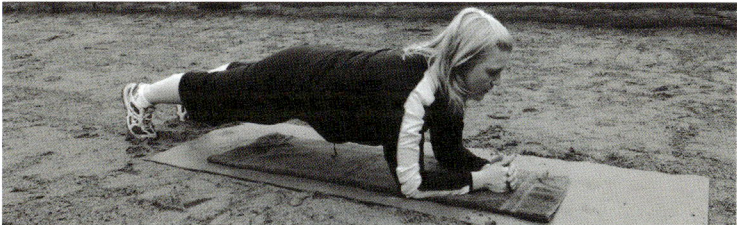

PLANK: Place elbows on the ground, under armpits (hands in prayer position) with back and legs perfectly straight. Weight is on your toes and elbows. If this hurts your lower back, tip pelvis forward and tighten stomach. If it still hurts, go on your knees.

workout 12 lower

1 mile run + basics + sprints + lower = kick ass workout

Not many surprises in today's workout. Make sure you go all the way down with the individual lunges, especially as you get tired. You can do it!

EXERCISE	YOUR GOAL	TIME LIMIT	How many did you do?
Alternate between exercises 1 and 2.			
1. LUNGE WALKS	7 x 10	10 mins	
2. JUMP SQUATS	7 x 10	5 mins	
Alternate between exercises 3 and 4.			
3. INDIVIDUAL LUNGE	3 x 10 each side	9 mins	
4. KNEE UPS	3 x 10 each side	10 mins	

Remember to eat before working out – you need the energy to burn maximum calories and train at 85%. Without food, your blood sugar drops and it's tough to train hard because your body looks to your muscles for stored glycogen.

your exercises today

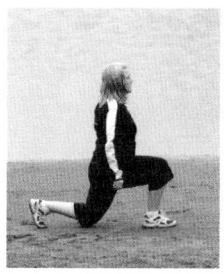 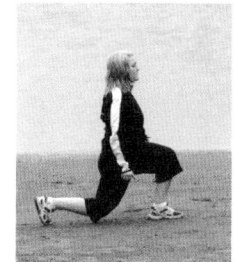

LUNGE WALKS: Take a big step forward, and lower yourself down so that your front leg is horizontal. Create a square and make sure the knees never go over your toes.

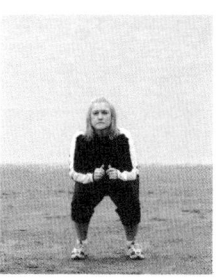 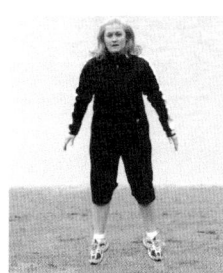

JUMP SQUATS: Keep your feet wide, torso strong, head up, and make sure the knees never go over your toes in the squat position. Stick your butt out and jump up, fully extended.

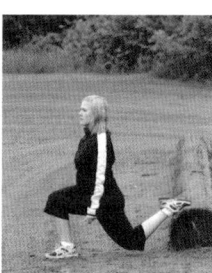 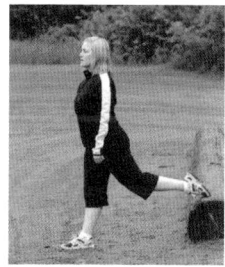

INDIVIDUAL LUNGE: Left foot should be far enough forward to allow yourself to sink deeply down without the knee going over the toe. Bend the right leg and sink as low as you can. You might want to hold onto your knee.

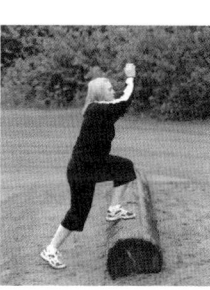 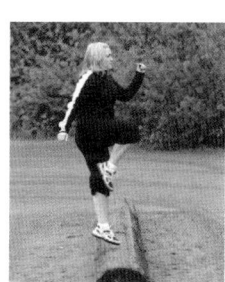 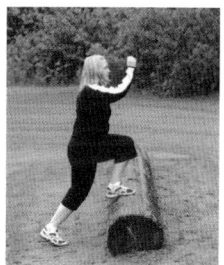

KNEE UPS: Plant right foot firmly on log or bench. Drive left leg up to chest explosively, tap down on ground and drive it right back up. Use your arms to balance yourself.

workout 13 upper

1 mile run + basics + sprints + upper = kick ass workout

In addition to your workout today, you will be measured. For accuracy this should be the same person who measured you in week one.

Write your results. See! The hard work is paying off!

WARM UP JOG,	5 mins
Today you're getting measured! See page 64	
Test your fitness again. Look how far you've come in 4 weeks! See page 66	
BICEP CURLS	3 x 25 reps
LUNGES	3 x 25 reps

Cravings for salt? Just like smoking, food addictions are tough to quit. Sweat out excess salt through daily exercise and eat more potassium. Try protein shakes (with banana, blue-green algae, yogurt) canned fish, olives, tomatoes, seaweed-based products and celery.

your exercises today

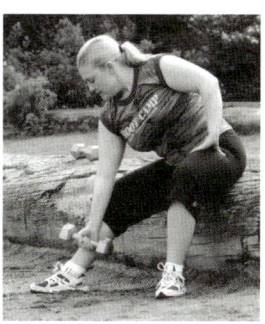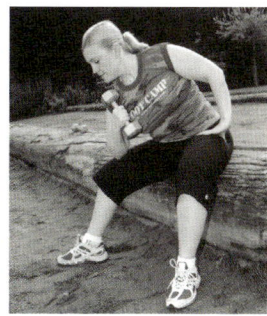

BICEP CURL: Sit down with your calf on an angle, elbow is in the groove of your knee. Curl up on an angle, into your arm pit. Twist your wrist at the top and relax your fingers.

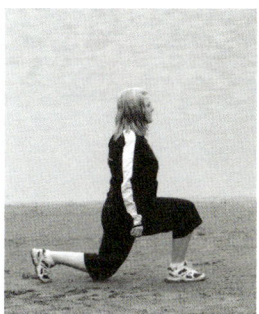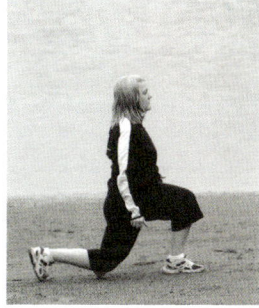

LUNGE WALKS: Take a big step forward, and lower yourself down so that your front leg is horizontal. Create a square and make sure the knees never go over your toes.

workout 14 core

1 mile run + basics + sprints + core = kick ass workout

You're over the hardest part – just stick with it and don't let procrastination interfere with your motivation. You know you're better than that!

EXERCISE	YOUR GOAL	TIME LIMIT	How many did you do?
Alternate between exercises 1 and 2.			
1. BICYCLE	3 x 10 each side	2 mins	
2. BOMBER CRUNCH	3 x 20	8 mins	
Alternate between exercises 3 and 4.			
3. SLOW SWIM	4 x 15	3 mins	
4. FLUTTER KICK	3 x 50	4 mins	

Wish your friends, boyfriend or co-workers would shape up with you? Instead of trying to change them, change yourself. Make new friends who are also trying to shape up (online, at the gym, in the nutrition store) and boost your chances of success!

your exercises today

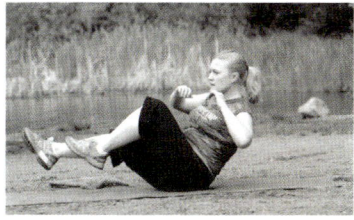 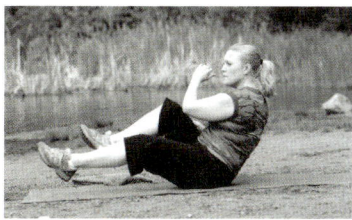

BICYCLE: Lie on back, hands behind head comfortably, legs straight. Bend knees up to chest, opposite leg outstretched. Twist torso to touch right elbow on left knee, then switch. If this puts strain on your back, bend knees up to chest (feet close to butt).

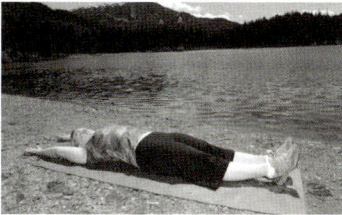 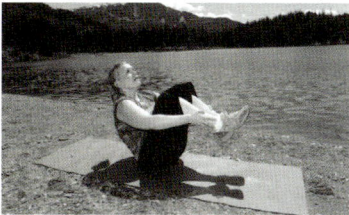

BOMBER CRUNCH: Lie on back, arms straight and outstretched over the head, legs on the ground. Throw arms up explosively and bend knees in a cannon ball, touching hands to ankles. Collapse back to starting position and do it all again.

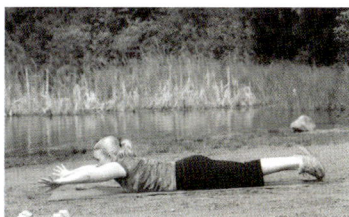 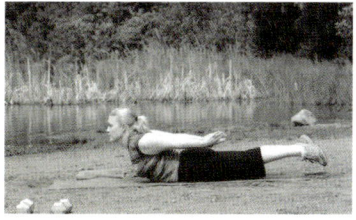

SLOW SWIM: Lie on stomach, hands in front of you and feet off the ground. Squeeze arms back slowly in a breast stroke swimming movement and squeeze shoulder blades together, holding until it hurts!, lifting feet off the ground when your arms come back.

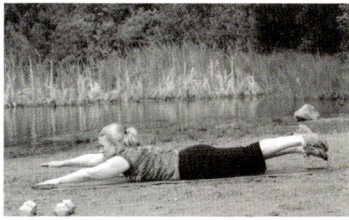 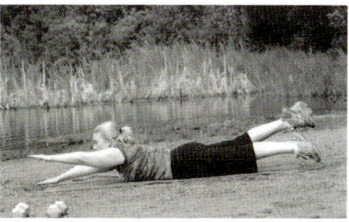

FLUTTER KICK: Lie on stomach, lift right arm up and left leg up at the same time, keeping left arm and right leg off the ground. Switch. Remember to breath! Keep head down if this aggravates your nexk.

workout 15 lower

1 mile run + basics + sprints + lower = kick ass workout

Ready for another big one? Lower is always tough.

See if you can convince a friend to join you!

EXERCISE	YOUR GOAL	TIME LIMIT	How many did you do?
Alternate between exercises 1 and 2.			
1. TELEMARK LUNGE (telemark skiing)	3 x 20	5 mins	
2. LUNGE WALK	3 x 20	4 mins	
Alternate between exercises 3 and 4.			
3. SQUATS	5 x 10	2 mins	
4. JUMP SQUATS	5 x 10	5 mins	

 I often hear…"I'm doing my cardio, but can't seem to get the weight off". Truth is, most exercisers achieve the target duration yet train under their target zone. Solution? Get a heart rate monitor and find your magic number: subtract your age from 220 and multiply by 70 to 85%.

your exercises today

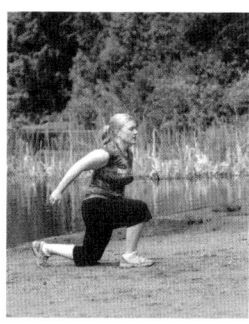 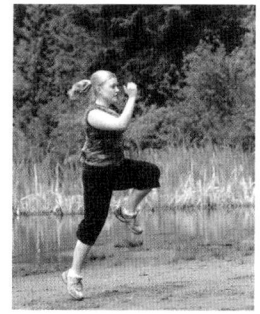

TELEMARK LUNGES: Similar to regular lunges, except harder! Explode up, driving one knee up to your chest. Travel vertically, not horizontally. Make sure when you lunge, your knee does not go over toe. Keep torso straight and drive arms to help balance yourself.

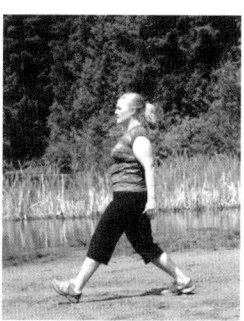 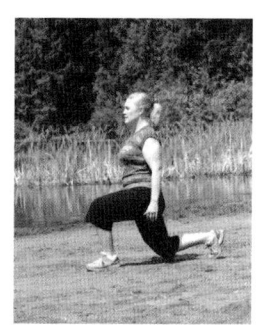

LUNGE WALKS: Take a big step forward, and lower yourself down so that your front leg is horizontal. Create a square and make sure the knees never go over your toes.

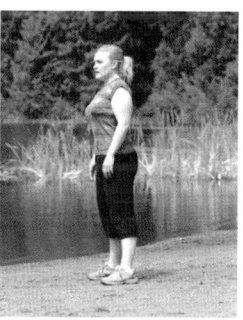 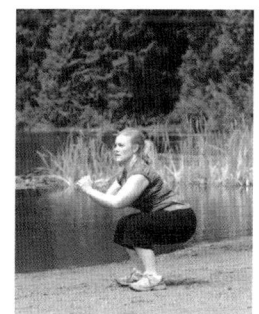

SQUATS: Keep your feet wide, stick your butt right out and head up. Sink down until thighs are horizontal to the ground, sticking your butt out and making sure knees never go over your toes. Breathe out as you come up.

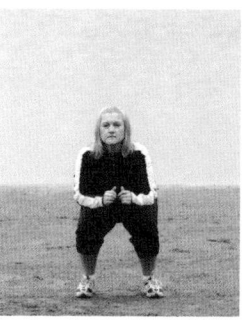 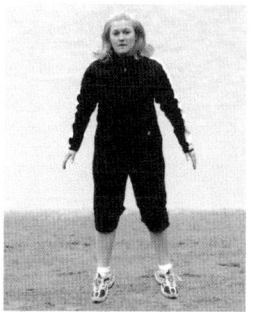

JUMP SQUATS: Keep your feet wide, torso strong, head up, and don't let knees never go over your toes.

workout 16 upper

1 mile run + basics + sprints + upper = kick ass workout

Come on!!!!!!!!! Yes YOU!!!!

EXERCISE	YOUR GOAL	TIME LIMIT	How many did you do?
Alternate between exercises 1 and 2.			
1. OVERHEAD SHOULDER RAISE	2 x 10 each side	7 mins	
2. INDIVIDUAL SHOULDER RAISE	2 x 20 each side	2 mins	
Alternate between exercises 3 and 4.			
3. BICEP CURLS	3 x 25 each side	4 mins	
4. TRICEP DIPS	3 x 25	2 mins	

Lighten up your eating patterns one meal at a time; for lunch today, try flavouring foods with fresh salsa, lemon, chutney, herbs and spices!

your exercises today

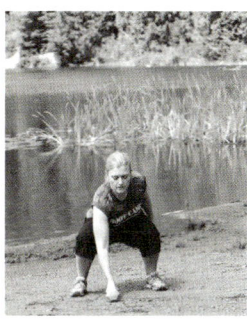 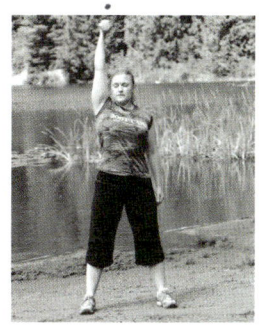

OVERHEAD SHOULDER RAISE: Stand in squat position, left hand in the small of lower back, torso strong, head and chest up. Squat down, touch the weight to the ground, up above your head, back to armpit and to the ground. You'll still be sore in your legs from Wednesday?

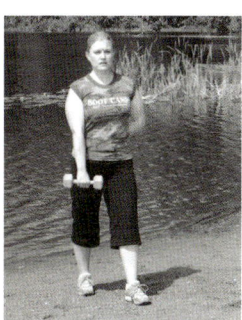 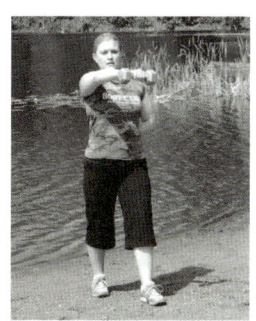

INDIVIDUAL SHOULDER RAISE: Stand with right leg forward, lifting left arm up to shoulder height. Bend arm and feel your shoulder moving in isolation. Keep torso still, bend knees slightly.

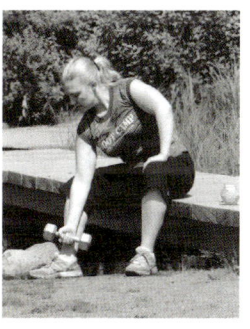 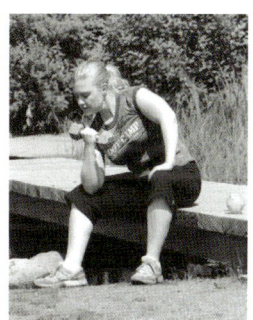

BICEP CURL: You know the position - calf is on an angle, elbow is in the groove of your knee. Curl up on an angle, into your arm pit.

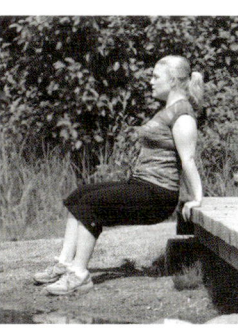 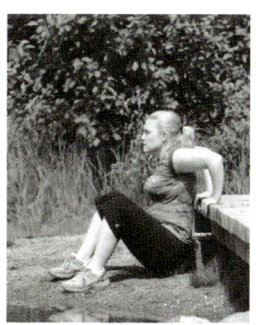

TRICEP DIP: Sit down and place hands beside your butt, elbows directly behind you. Feet are firmly on the ground, knees bent and toes relaxed. Dip down so that the backs of your arms are horizontal to the ground, forearms vertical.

workout 17 core

1 mile run + basics + sprints + core = kick ass workout

We've all got our weaknesses. The plank might be yours........most recruits
HATE this exercise. But keep at it - the results will be worth it!

EXERCISE	YOUR GOAL	TIME LIMIT	How many did you do?
Alternate between exercises 1 and 2.			
1. FLUTTER CRUNCH	3 x 25 crunches	5 mins	
2. PLANK	3 x 60 secs	3 mins	
Alternate between exercises 3 and 4.			
3. SLOW SWIM	4 x 15	2 mins	
4. SUPERMAN	4 x 15	2 mins	

 Caffeinate your workouts! Caffeine releases calcium, letting you run faster as it increases the strength of your muscle contractions. It also delays the brain's perception of feeling pain and fatigue, meaning you can kick ass in your workouts for longer.

your exercises today

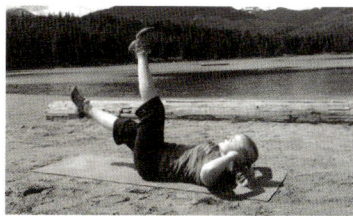 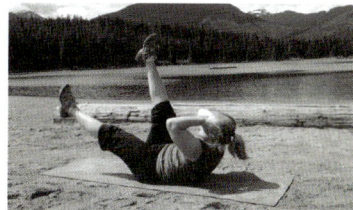

FLUTTER CRUNCH: Lie on back, hands comfortably behind head, legs vertical. Alternate legs back and forth, only going down as far as you can keep your lower back on the ground. Don't let hip flexors click. Crunch upwards aggressively every time your right leg comes up (not side to side) bringing shoulders off the ground.

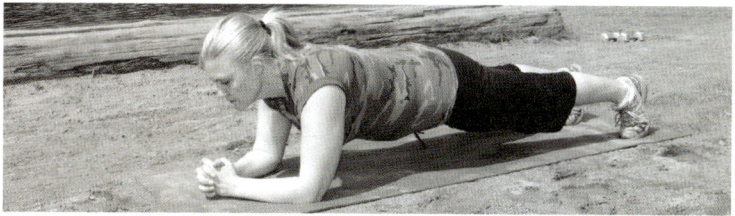

PLANK: Place elbows on the ground directly under armpits (hands in prayer position) with back and legs perfectly straight. Weight is on your toes and elbows.

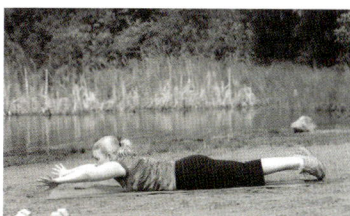 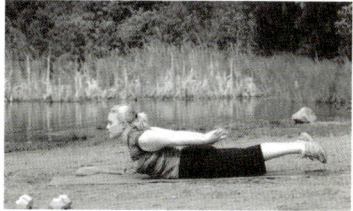

SLOW SWIM: Lie on stomach, hands in front of you and feet on the ground. Squeeze arms back slowly in a breast stroke swimming movement and squeeze shoulder blades together, holding until it hurts, lifting feet off the ground.

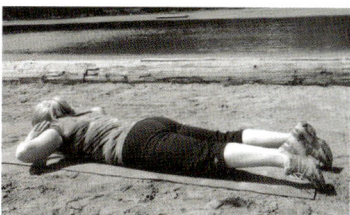 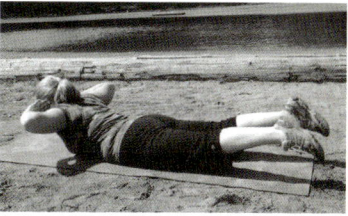

SUPERMAN: Lie on stomach, arms outstretched in flying position or under your chin, legs straight and off the ground. Lift up chest to maximum extension and pulse up and down 3 inches.

workout 18 lower

1 mile run + basics + sprints + lower = kick ass workout

Have a look at yourself in the mirror. See how strong you have become, and healthy you look. Appreciate what you have become, and the strength you've shown getting this far!

EXERCISE	YOUR GOAL	TIME LIMIT	How many did you do?
Alternate between exercises 1 and 2.			
1. LUNGE WALKS	10 x 10	8 mins	
2. SQUATS	10 x 10	4 mins	
Alternate between exercises 3 and 4.			
3. KNEE UPS	3 x 10 each side	10 mins	
4. INDIVIDUAL LUNGE	3 x 10 each side	8 mins	

 Those who keep their fitness in perspective have higher body confidence, happiness and patience than their friends that overdo it. Find what fits your life.

your exercises today

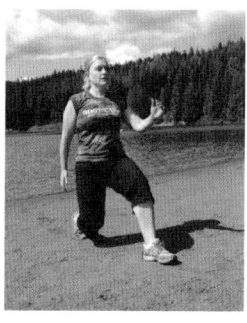 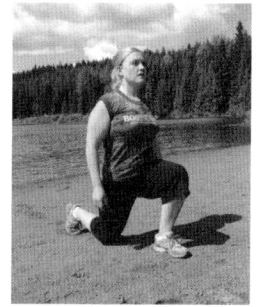

LUNGE WALKS: Take a big step forward, and lower yourself down so that your front leg is horizontal. Create a square and make sure the knees stay behind your toes.

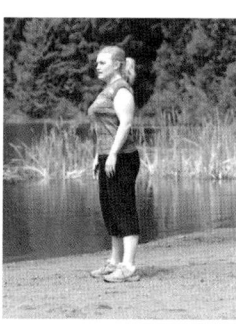 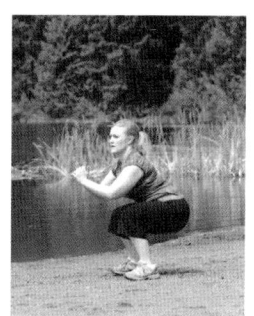

SQUATS: Keep your feet wide, stick your butt right out (keeping torso strong) and head up. Sink down until thighs are horizontal to the ground, knees behind your toes. Breathe out as you come up.

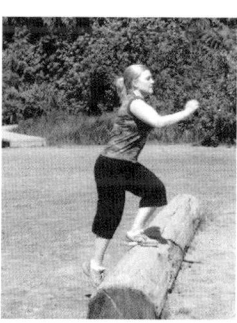 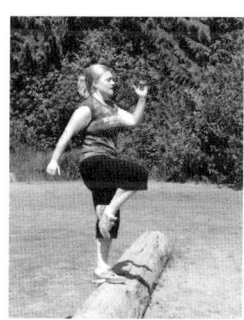

KNEE UPS: Plant right foot firmly on log or bench. Drive left leg up to chest explosively, tap down on the ground, drive it right back up. Use your arms to balance yourself.

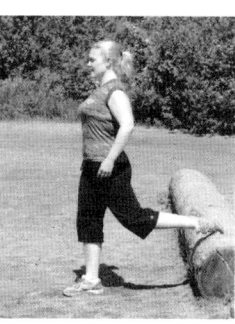 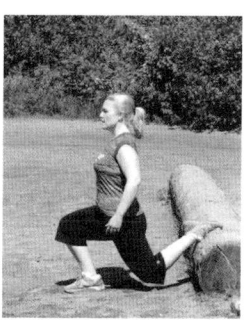

INDIVIDUAL LUNGE: Place right foot directly behind you, with knee bent and torso straight. Left foot should be far enough forward to allow yourself to sink deeply down without the knee going over the toe. Bend the right leg and sink as low as you can.

workout 19 upper

1 mile run + basics + sprints + upper = kick ass workout

The biceps will be much stronger now than they were six weeks ago.
If you feel up to it, try lifting with a heavier weight for a few reps.

EXERCISE	YOUR GOAL	TIME LIMIT	How many did you do?
Alternate between exercises 1 and 2.			
1. SHOULDER PRESS	3 x 20	6 mins	
2. LATERAL RAISE	3 x 10	4 mins	
Alternate between exercises 3 and 4.			
3. BICEP CURL	3 x 25 each side	6 mins	
4. TRICEP PRESS	3 x 25	3 mins	

 You wouldn't let your dog spend a day without exercise, why allow yourself to? Eat right and live well: self-respect is about knowing you are putting in your best effort.

your exercises today

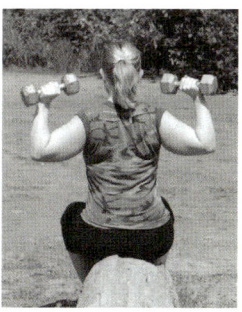 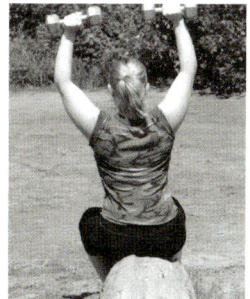

SHOULDER PRESS: Push weight up until arms are straight. Bring down, squeezing shoulder blades - elbows as low down your sides as possible.

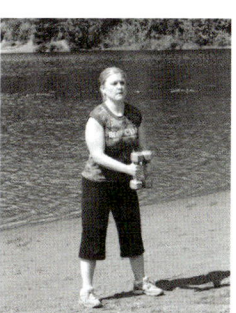 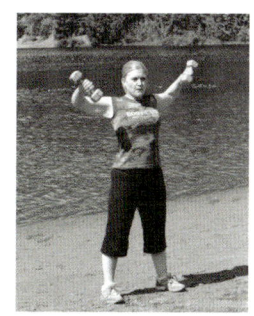

LATERAL RAISE: Stand with ankles, knees and hips flexed. Push off toes and raise arms to the side, leading with your elbows. Keep hands at elbow level. Squeeze shoulder blades as you come up, chest as you come down.

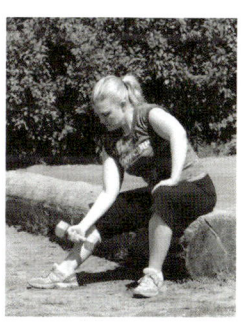 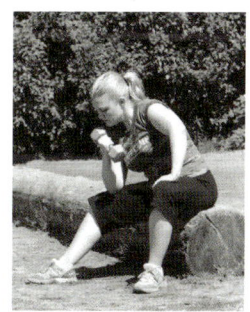

BICEP CURL: Sit with calf on an angle, elbow in the groove of your knee. Curl up on an angle, into your arm pit. Twist wrist at the top.

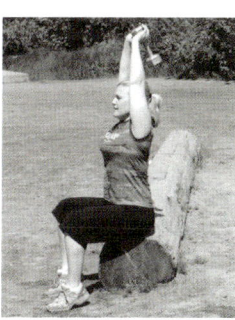 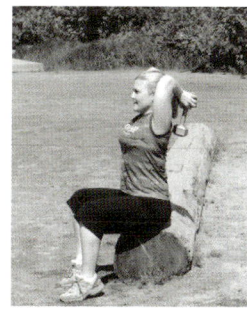

TRICEP PRESS: Sit down, feet firmly planted, torso slightly forwards. Start with weight touching the back of your spine, elbows over your ears. Push up weight until arms are straight. Make sure you always keep elbows close to head.

workout 20 core

1 mile run + basics + sprints + core = kick ass workout

Keep in mind, you don't have to do the entire workout at once.

If your day is busy do the run and basics in the morning. and the other exercises after work.

EXERCISE	YOUR GOAL	TIME LIMIT	How many did you do?
Alternate between exercises 1 and 2.			
1. FLUTTER CRUNCH	3 x 50 crunches	5 mins	
2. BICYCLE	3 x 25 each side	3 mins	
Alternate between exercises 3 and 4.			
3. BOMBER CRUNCH	3 x 20	8 mins	
4. SLOW SWIM	3 x 20	3 mins	

Those who see the funny side of life might find more power to stay fit! Laughing boosts tolerance to pain and increases your immunity, which in turn, jolts energy levels.

your exercises today

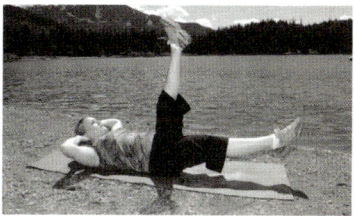 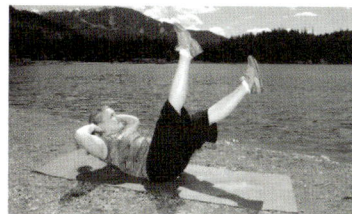

FLUTTER CRUNCH: Lie on back, hands comfortably behind head, legs vertical. Alternate legs back and forth, only going down as far as you can keep your lower back on the ground. Don't let hip flexors click. Crunch upwards aggressively in sync with right leg coming up (not side to side) bringing shoulders off the ground.

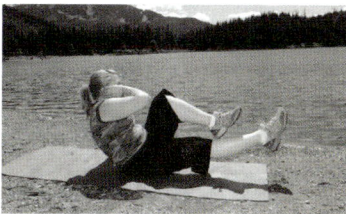 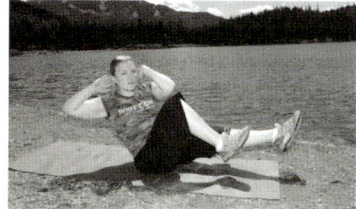

BICYCLE: Hands behind head, legs straight. Bend knees up to chest, opposite leg outstretched. Twist torso to touch right elbow on left knee, then switch. If this starts to work your legs or back, bring knees up to chest and keep feet closer to butt.

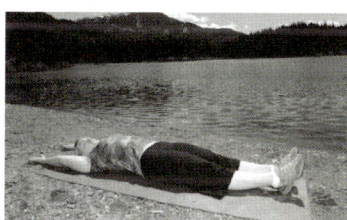 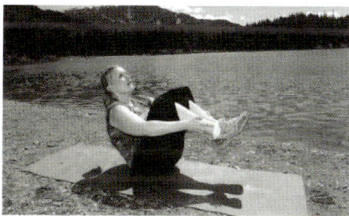

BOMBER CRUNCH: Lie on back, arms straight and outstretched over the head, legs on the ground. Throw arms up explosively and bend knees in a cannon ball, touching hands to ankles. Collapse back to starting position and do it all again.

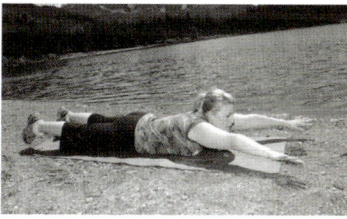 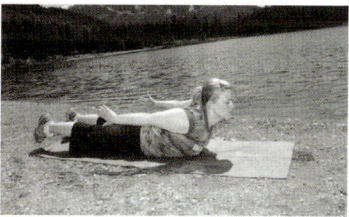

SLOW SWIM: Lie on stomach, hands in front of you and feet off the ground. Squeeze arms back slowly in a breast stroke swimming movement and squeeze shoulder blades together, holding until it hurts!

workout 21 lower

1 mile run + basics + sprints + lower = kick ass workout

Today we push the traditional lunge to the next level.....! You can do it!

Nice work!

EXERCISE	YOUR GOAL	TIME LIMIT	How many did you do?
Alternate between exercises 1 and 2.			
1. TELEMARK LUNGE	4 x 20	5 mins	
2. SUMO SQUAT	4 x 20	5 mins	
Alternate between exercises 3 and 4.			
3. SIDE LUNGE	2 x 10 each side	5 mins	
4. SUMO JUMP SQUAT	3 x 10	2 mins	

Get hooked on exercise for reasons beyond weight loss and you'll make it a way of life. Twenty years from now, you'll remember the summer you fell in love with mountain biking or became a rafting instructor – not what you looked like on the beach!

your exercises today

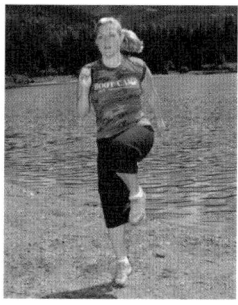 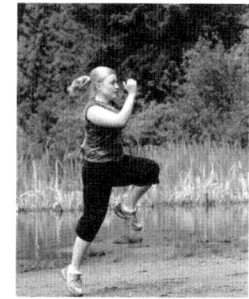

TELEMARK LUNGES: Similar to regular lunges, except harder! Explode up, driving one knee up to your chest. Travel vertically, not horizontally. Keep knee behind toe. Keep torso straight and drive arms to help balance yourself.

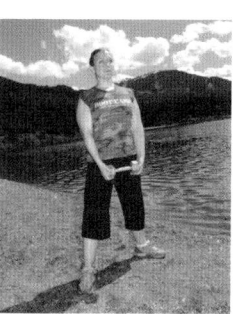 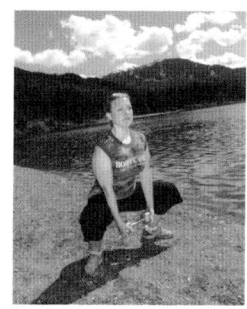

SUMO SQUAT: Stand with feet wide apart, toes pointing as outwards as your flexibility will allow without losing balance. Push pelvis forward and sink down as far as you can, keeping torso straight. Feel your inner thighs! Holding the weight is optional.

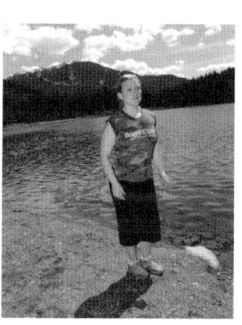 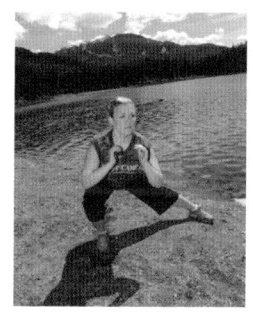

SIDE LUNGE: Start in standing position, take a big step out to the side (slightly in front of you) and sink down into a side lunge. Keep knee directly above your foot, without going over toes. Elbows should be on either side of the knee holding your weight.

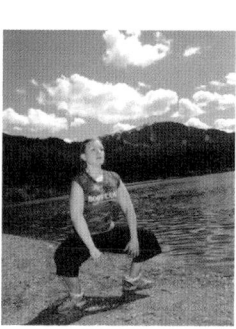 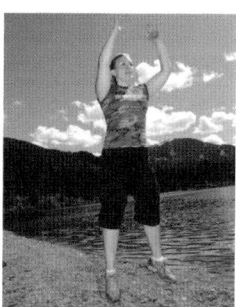

SUMO JUMP SQUAT: Exactly the same as the Sumo Squat except when you come up, jump!

workout 22 upper

1 mile run + basics + sprints + upper = kick ass workout

If you've got this far, you're almost there!

EXERCISE	YOUR GOAL	TIME LIMIT	How many did you do?
Alternate between exercises 1 and 2.			
1. SHOULDER PRESS	3 x 25	4 mins	
2. INDIVIDUAL SHOULDER RAISE	2 x 25 each side	6 mins	
Alternate between exercises 3 and 4.			
3. UPRIGHT ROW	2 x 25	4 min	
4. PUNCH THRU	2 x 25 each side	4 mins	

 Stoke your metabolic fire before workouts by eating around 150-200 calories worth of carb-dense mini meals, pre session. Play with combinations to find your favorite – try peanut butter on whole wheat toast, a soy latte or some yogurt.

your exercises today

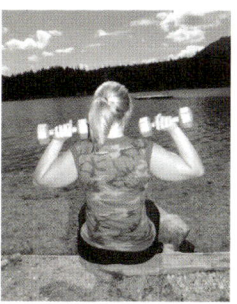 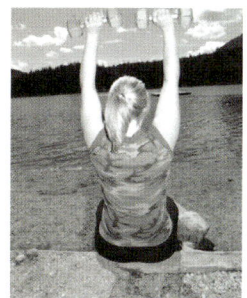

SHOULDER PRESS: Push up until arms are straight, twisting wrists slightly at the top. Bring elbows down low, squeezing shoulder blades. Push back up using your shoulder strength.

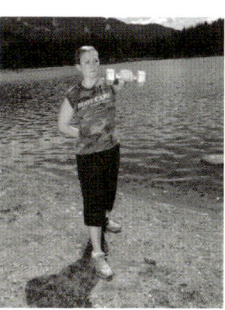 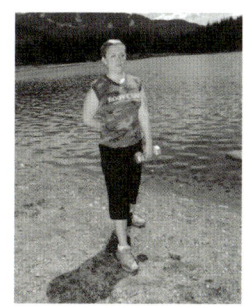

INDIVIDUAL SHOULDER RAISE: Stand with right leg forward in athletic position, lifting left arm up to shoulder height. Bend arm and work shoulder in isolation. Keep torso still, bend knees slightly.

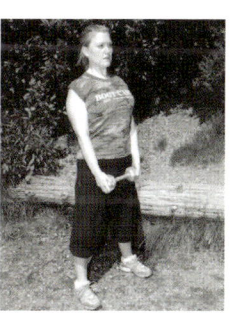 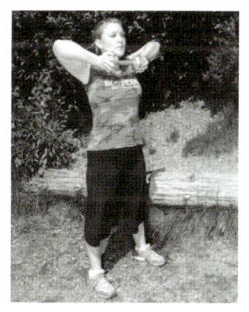

UPRIGHT ROW: Stand athletically with feet shoulder-width apart. Hold each end of the weight, and lift up to touch top of chest with weight. Lead with the elbows, squeezing shoulder blades as you come up. Avoid rolling or moving wrists at any stage of this exercise.

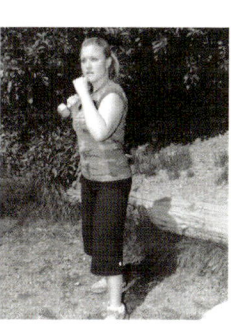 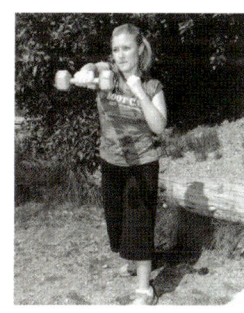

PUNCH THRU: Stand with left leg forward (knees bent) and right hand holding weight close to your face. Keeping elbow close to body, punch out aggressively, twisting wrist at the impact point (the end). Snap back weight to your face. Don't let your hands drop!

workout 23 core

1 mile run + basics + sprints + core = kick ass workout

With the weekend off and the end in sight, motivation should be at an all-time high. But don't relax just yet! It's not over till it's over.

EXERCISE	YOUR GOAL	TIME LIMIT	How many did you do?
Alternate between exercises 1 and 2.			
1. BOMBER CRUNCH	3 x 25	5 mins	
2. V-UPS	3 x 25	5 mins	
Alternate between exercises 3 and 4.			
3. FLUTTER CRUNCH	3 x 50	5 mins	
4. FLUTTER KICK	3 x 50	2 mins	

 When you put in your best effort, it shows. Pride is a beautiful thing!

your exercises today

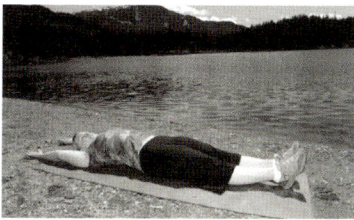 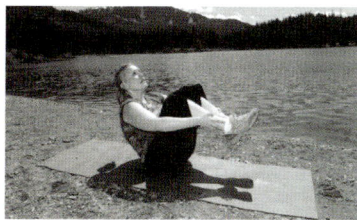

BOMBER CRUNCH: Lie on back, arms straight and outstretched over the head, legs on the ground. Throw arms up explosively and bend knees in a cannon ball, touching hands to ankles. Collapse back to starting position and do it all again.

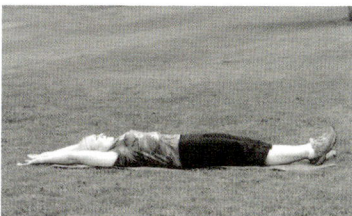 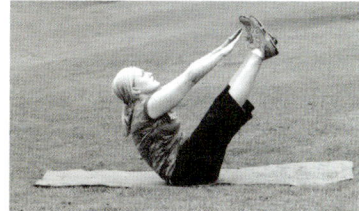

V-UPS: Exactly the same as the bomber crunch, except with straight legs - and even harder! Throw arms up agressively so the torso comes up quicker than the legs. Aim to touch toes, like a divers pike.

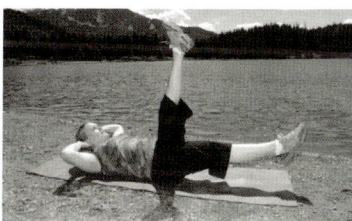 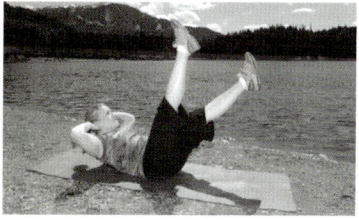

FLUTTER CRUNCH: Lie on back, hands comfortably behind head, legs vertical. Alternate legs back and forth, only going down as far as you can keep your lower back on the ground. Don't let hip flexors click. Crunch upwards agressively in sync with right leg coming up (not side to side) bringing shoulders off the ground.

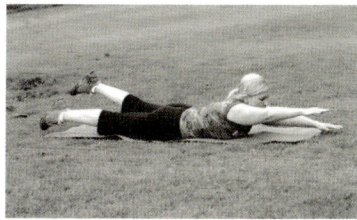 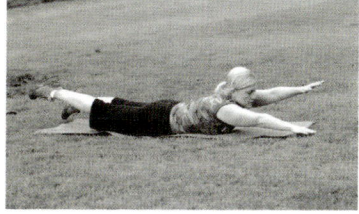

FLUTTER KICK: Lie on stomach, lift right arm up and left leg up at the same time, keeping left arm and right leg off the ground. Switch. Remember to breathe! Keep head down if this aggravates your neck. Keep hands and feet off the ground.

workout 24 testing

Congratulations! You've kicked ass!

WARM UP JOG,	5 mins
Today you're getting measured! See page 64	
Test your fitness again. Look how far you've come in 8 weeks! See page 66	
BICEP CURLS	3 x 25 reps
LUNGES	3 x 25 reps

 Wanting what you don't have is a sure way to spoil what you do. What you have right now was once something you hoped for!

your exercises today

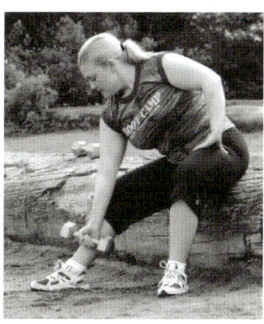 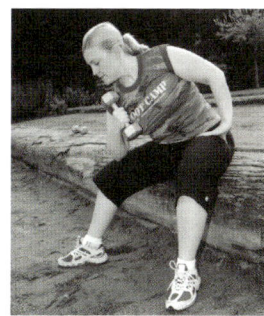

BICEP CURL: Sit down with your calf on an angle, elbow is in the groove of your knee. Curl up on an angle, into your arm pit. Twist your wrist at the top and relax your fingers.

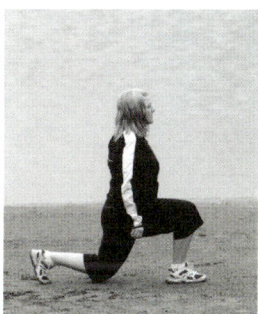 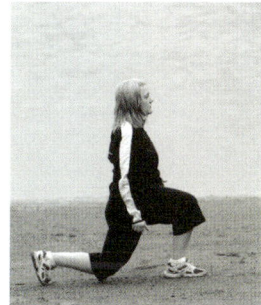

LUNGE WALKS: Take a big step forward, and lower yourself down so that your front leg is horizontal. Create a square and make sure the knees never go over your toes.

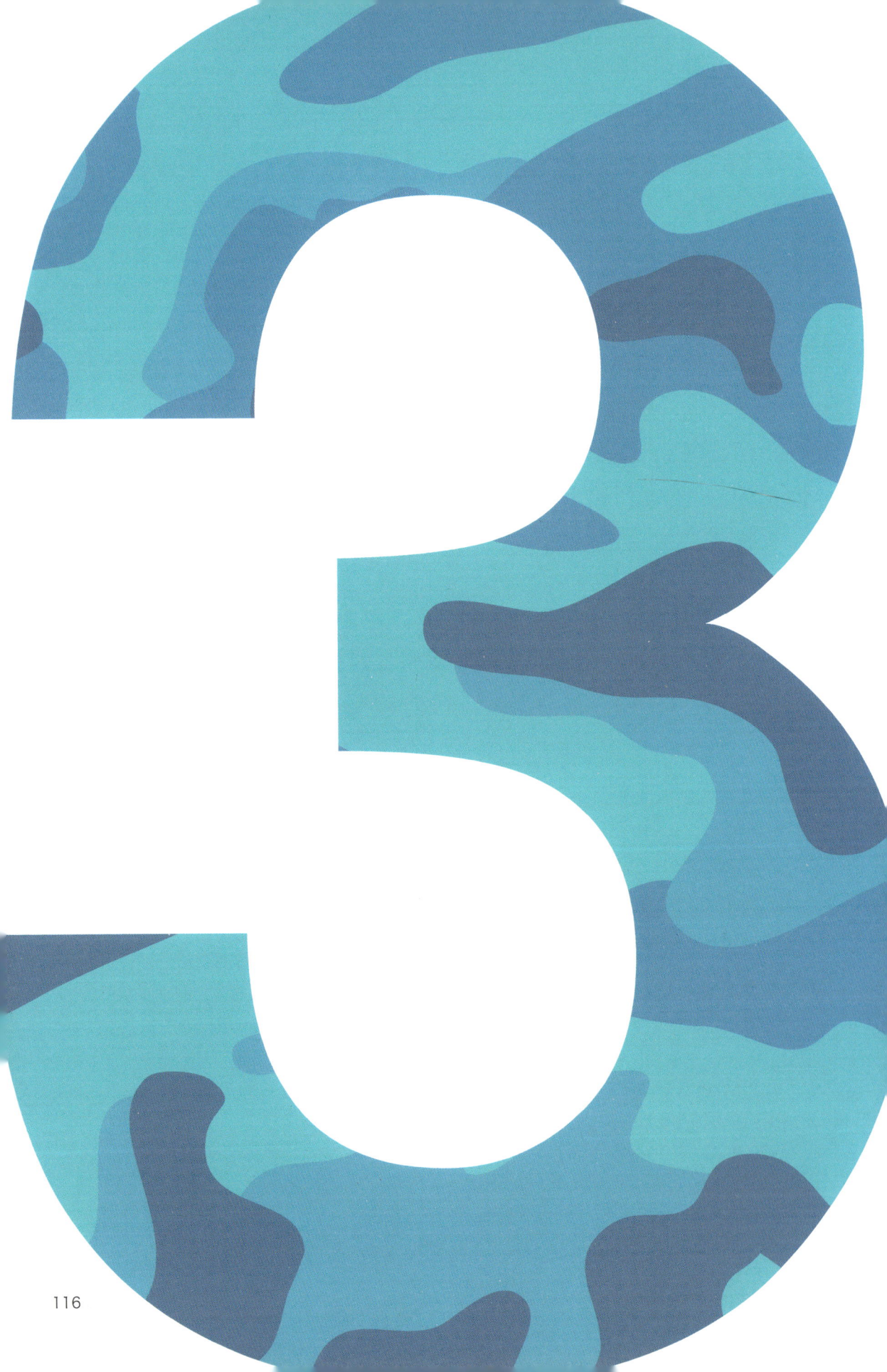

8 week training journal

week 1 _____ to _____

goals:

day 1

weight

hours slept:

esitmated calories eaten:

water:

workout:

Losing weight is like training for the Olympics. You'll face defeat, you'll face victory – but at the end of the day, you'll face the toughest critic....yourself.

day 2

weight ⬭

hours slept:

esitmated calories eaten:

water:

workout:

---

day 3

weight ⬭

hours slept:

esitmated calories eaten:

water:

workout:

day 4

weight 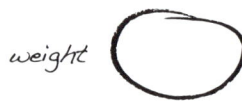 hours slept:

esitmated calories eaten: water:

workout:

---

day 5

weight 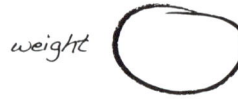 hours slept:

esitmated calories eaten: water:

workout:

day 6

weight ( )　　　　　　hours slept:

esitmated calories eaten:　　　　　　water:

workout:

---

day 7

weight ( )　　　　　　hours slept:

esitmated calories eaten:　　　　　　water:

workout:

week 2 _____ to _____

goals:

day 8

weight ◯   hours slept:

esitmated calories eaten: water:

workout:

Want to kick ass? Check your attitude, belief and enthusiasm.
The decision to train is made emotionally, then put into action logically.
Change your mind and success will be yours.

day 9

weight ( )   hours slept:

esitmated calories eaten: water:

workout:

---

day 10

weight ( )   hours slept:

esitmated calories eaten: water:

workout:

day 11

weight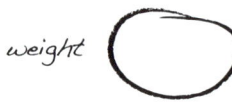

hours slept:

esitmated calories eaten:

water:

workout:

---

day 12

weight

hours slept:

esitmated calories eaten:

water:

workout:

day 13

weight ⬭   hours slept:

esitmated calories eaten: water:

workout:

---

day 14

weight ⬭   hours slept:

esitmated calories eaten: water:

workout:

week 3 _____ to _____

goals:

day 15

weight ⬭

hours slept:

esitmated calories eaten:

water:

workout:

"Every day, in some way, I am kicking ass." Positive self-talk is an important part of moving towards your goals. Say it, see it, do it!

day 16

weight ◯   hours slept:

esitmated calories eaten: water:

workout:

---

day 17

weight ◯   hours slept:

esitmated calories eaten: water:

workout:

day 18

weight 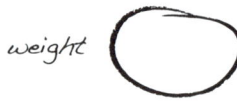   hours slept:

esitmated calories eaten: water:

workout:

---

day 19

weight 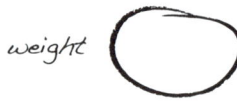   hours slept:

esitmated calories eaten: water:

workout:

day 20

weight ( )   hours slept:

esitmated calories eaten: water:

workout:

---

day 21

weight ( )   hours slept:

esitmated calories eaten: water:

workout:

week 4 _____ to _____

goals:

day 22

weight ⬭   hours slept:

esitmated calories eaten: water:

workout:

Reaching the top of your game takes MONTHS of kick ass workouts, sweat, sacrifices, endorphin and dedication to your diet. You want it?
Go get it! There are no shortcuts.

day 23

weight ⬭

hours slept:

esitmated calories eaten:

water:

workout:

---

day 24

weight ⬭

hours slept:

esitmated calories eaten:

water:

workout:

day 25

weight 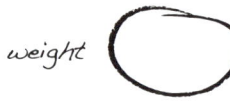   hours slept:

esitmated calories eaten: water:

workout:

---

day 26

weight 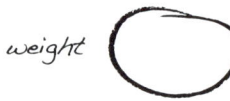   hours slept:

esitmated calories eaten: water:

workout:

day 27

weight ⬭

hours slept:

esitmated calories eaten:

water:

workout:

---

day 28

weight ⬭

hours slept:

esitmated calories eaten:

water:

workout:

K!CK ASS WORKOUTS K!CK ASS
ORKOUTS K!CK ASS WORKOUTS K!CK ASS WO
OUTS K!CK ASS WORKOUTS K!CK ASS A

week 5 _____ to _____

goals:

day 29

weight ◯   hours slept:

esitmated calories eaten: water:

workout:

Don't try to be better than others when you're working out.
Try to be better than yourself.

day 30

weight ◯   hours slept:

esitmated calories eaten: water:

workout:

---

day 31

weight ◯   hours slept:

esitmated calories eaten: water:

workout:

day 32

weight 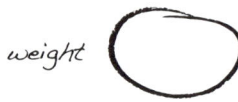　　　　hours slept:

esitmated calories eaten:　　　　water:

workout:

---

day 33

weight 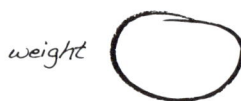　　　　hours slept:

esitmated calories eaten:　　　　water:

workout:

day 34

weight ⬭   hours slept:

esitmated calories eaten: water:

workout:

---

day 35

weight ⬭   hours slept:

esitmated calories eaten: water:

workout:

week 6 _____ to _____

goals:

day 36

weight ◯

hours slept:

esitmated calories eaten:

water:

workout:

Train like you're an athlete and you'll help yourself become one. We all grow differently, but our roots come from the same place. Imagine, believe, become!

day 37

weight ( )

hours slept:

esitmated calories eaten:

water:

workout:

---

day 38

weight ( )

hours slept:

esitmated calories eaten:

water:

workout:

day 39

weight 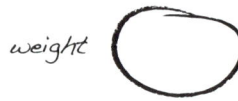   hours slept:

esitmated calories eaten: water:

workout:

---

day 40

weight ◯   hours slept:

esitmated calories eaten: water:

workout:

day 41

weight ⬭   hours slept:

esitmated calories eaten: water:

workout:

---

day 42

weight ⬭   hours slept:

esitmated calories eaten: water:

workout:

week 7 _____ to _____

goals:

day 43

weight ⬭   hours slept:

esitmated calories eaten: water:

workout:

The best way to predict the future is to create it – what we are is a result of what we have become. So get out there and make the most of yourself and this awesome day!

day 44

weight ⬭

hours slept:

esitmated calories eaten:

water:

workout:

---

day 45

weight ⬭

hours slept:

esitmated calories eaten:

water:

workout:

day 46

weight 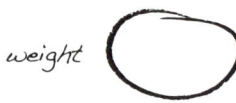   hours slept:

esitmated calories eaten: water:

workout:

---

day 47

weight 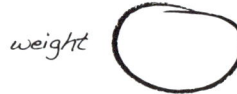   hours slept:

esitmated calories eaten: water:

workout:

KICK ASS WORKOUTS

day 48

weight ⬭   hours slept:

esitmated calories eaten: water:

workout:

---

day 49

weight ⬭   hours slept:

esitmated calories eaten: water:

workout:

week 8 _____ to _____

goals:

day 50

weight ⭕   hours slept:

esitmated calories eaten: water:

workout:

*Any exerciser can become an athlete when they start thinking like one.
It's only once you leave your disabling beliefs at home that you can elevate
your perception of what you can achieve!*

day 51

weight ⬭   hours slept:

esitmated calories eaten: water:

workout:

---

day 52

weight ⬭   hours slept:

esitmated calories eaten: water:

workout:

day 53

weight 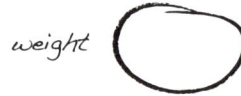   hours slept:

esitmated calories eaten: water:

workout:

---

day 54

weight 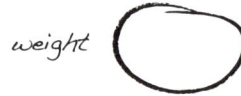   hours slept:

esitmated calories eaten: water:

workout: